THE
FACTS
of
HORMONE THERAPY
for Menopausal Women

THE FACTS

of

HORMONE THERAPY

for Menopausal Women

David W. Sturdee

Solihull Hospital, Solihull, UK

The Parthenon Publishing Group

International Publishers in Medicine, Science & Technology

A CRC PRESS COMPANY

BOCA RATON   LONDON   NEW YORK   WASHINGTON, D.C.

Published in the USA by
The Parthenon Publishing Group
345 Park Avenue South, 10th Floor
New York, NY 10010, USA

Published in the UK and Europe by
The Parthenon Publishing Group Limited
23–25 Blades Court
Deodar Road
London SW15 2NU, UK

Library of Congress Cataloging-in-Publication Data

Sturdee, David W.
    The facts of hormone therapy for menopausal women/ David W. Sturdee.
       p. ; cm
    Includes bibliographical references and index.
    ISBN 1-85070-807-X (alk. paper)
    1. Menopause. 2. Menopause–Hormone therapy. 3. Middle aged women–Health and
    hygiene. I. Title
    [DNLM: 1. Estrogen Replacement Therapy. WP 522 S935F2003]
    RG186.S787 2003
    618.1'75061–dc21

                                         2003049877

British Library Cataloguing in Publication Data

Sturdee, David W.
    The facts of hormone therapy for menopausal women
    1. Menopause - Hormone therapy
    I. Title
    618.1'75'061

ISBN 1-85070-807-X

Composition by The Parthenon Publishing Group
Printed and bound by Butler & Tanner Ltd., Frome and London, UK

Contents

Introduction

It has long been known that acute menopausal symptoms such as hot flushes can be alleviated by estrogen replacement therapy. However, in the past decade, and particularly in the last 2 years, a wealth of research and development has been attempting to evaluate a possible preventative role of estrogen in the chronic diseases that beset the older woman, such as osteoporosis, heart disease and Alzheimer's disease. Moreover, the risks associated with hormone therapy (HT) are being quantified, and the few contraindications are well documented. The wide range of preparations, delivery routes and dosages now available enable most women to find a convenient form of treatment, free from side-effects. Traditionally, the term HRT has been used but this is not an appropriate term to cover all types of hormone treatment for menopausal women and, in keeping with recent proposals, the acronym HT will be used throughout this text[1,2].

The menopause is a natural and inevitable accompaniment of aging and women need to know what changes to expect, and to know what their options are for dealing with the far-reaching detrimental effects of declining estrogen levels. But the explosion of research has brought in its wake 'a sense of growing confusion amongst most women'[3] and the report in July 2002 from the Women's Health Initiative (WHI) in the USA has also provoked widespread anxiety about the safety of HT[4]. Women are interested in HT, but they are anxious and bewildered about side-effects and perceived risks[5]. At one general practitioner's surgery, over half of women classified as being at risk of osteoporosis declined treatment, but were unable to give well-founded reasons for their refusal[6].

This book is intended as a resource for family doctors and specialist nurses. It provides a concise account of recent advances in this exciting field, together with an outline of the evidence which informs current thinking. It is hoped that the information it contains will also prove useful to women interested in the up-to-date facts about HT. For the physician, prescription guidelines are included for women of different ages and clinical needs, highlighting the variety of treatment regimens currently in use. Primary care workers are well placed to provide evidence-based advice to help women decide whether they should use HT.

References

1. Sturdee DW, MacLennan AH. HT and HRT, that is the question? Time to change the terminology for hormone therapy. *Climacteric* 2003;6:1

2. NAMS Report. Amended report from the NAMS Advisory Panel on Postmenopausal Hormone Therapy. The North American Menopause Society. *Menopause* 2003;10:6–12

3. Leiblum SR, Swartzman LC. Women's attitudes towards the menopause: an update. *Maturitas* 1986;8:47–56

4. Writing Group for the Women's Health Initiative Investigators. Risks and benefits of estrogen plus progestin in healthy postmenopausal women. *J Am Med Assoc* 2002;288:321–33

5.   Draper J, Roland M. Perimenopausal women's views on taking HT to prevent osteoporosis. *Br Med J* 1990;300:786–8

6.   Wallace WA, Bruce VH, Elliot CA, MacPherson MBA, Scott BW. HT acceptability to Nottingham post-menopausal women with a risk factor for osteoporosis. *J R Soc Med* 1990;83:699–701

Chapter 1

HT in the 21st century

1.1 The life expectancy of women is increasing, while the age at which the menopause occurs remains unchanged

The average life expectancy of women in the Western world has now risen to 79 years, with increasing numbers living into their 80s and 90s (Tables 1.1 and 1.2). This upward trend will continue for the next 50 years. However, the average age at which the menopause occurs (51 in the developed world and a few years less elsewhere) has remained unaltered. This means that large numbers of women in the West will experience over

Table 1.1   Average female life expectancies since 1850

Year	Average female life expectancy (years)
1850	40
1900	55
1930	62
1955	73
2000	79

Table 1.2   Some population statistics

- At the age of 50 the life expectancy of women in the UK is 31.8 years

- In the United Kingdom, the number of women aged over 75 has risen from 2.6 million in 1991 to 2.8 million in 2001[2]

- The number of women aged over 85 is expected to rise by 50% in the next 20 years[3]

- In the United States, in 1997 there were 34 million people over the age of 65, representing 13% of the population. During the next 30 years, the number of over-65s will more than double, and the number of over-85s will triple[4]

- 70% of the over-85s are women[4]

- By the year 2050, 5% of the population will be 85 or over, and 42% of the then 65-year-olds will expect to live to the age of 90[4]

- In comparison, in 1997, the life expectancy in sub-Saharan Africa was 52 years, despite a 10% decrease in child mortality. In eight African countries, life expectancy has decreased by 3 years as a result of acquired immune deficiency syndrome (AIDS)[5]

one-third of their lives in the postmenopausal state and, increasingly, will be exposed to the major diseases characteristic of the elderly (Figure 1.1). This, in turn, will put an increasing burden on already stretched national health services. For example, osteoporosis alone costs the National Health Service in the UK nearly £1 billion per year[1].

It has long been known that hormone therapy (HT) relieves the acute symptoms caused by estrogen decline at the menopause. Recent studies have confirmed that HT reduces the incidence of osteoporosis and osteoporotic fractures, and possibly delays the onset of Alzheimer's disease. There is also considerable evidence from observational and laboratory studies for a preventive effect on coronary heart disease (CHD) and, until recently, this was considered to be a valid indication for HT. The widely published Women's Health Initiative (WHI) report from the USA in July

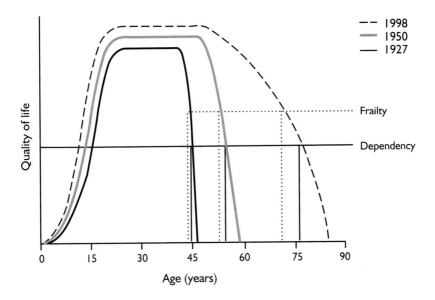

Figure 1.1

Average lifespan in 1927, 1950 and 1998. During the twentieth century, the increase in average lifespan resulted in longer periods of dependency. In 1999, the average lifespan was about 80 years and the most common causes of mortality were cancer, degenerative diseases, organ failure or immune deficiencies. Adapted from Lunenfeld B. Aging for men. In Studd J, ed. *The Management of the Menopause. The Millennium Review 2000.* Carnforth, UK: Parthenon Publishing, 2000

2002 has changed opinion and now the merits for CHD are less clear (see Chapter 6). Currently, less than 20% of women aged 50–65 years in the UK take HT and compliance is poor, with 25% of those who start treatment abandoning it within 6 months[6].

1.2 There are many different HT preparations to choose from

The wide range of HT preparations now available enables the clinician to customize the type, dose and delivery route of estrogen and progestogen to provide optimum therapeutic effect with minimal side-effects (see Appendix for available preparations). The needs of the older menopausal woman can be accommodated by the newer continuous combined regimens, which allow her to benefit from the protection afforded by estrogen, while remaining period-free.

Careful follow-up is necessary to help the patient through the early months, when treatment is most likely to be abandoned because of side-effects. The patient should understand that it is not unusual for a woman to try several formulations before settling on one which she finds acceptable[7]. Nevertheless, many women are happy with the first preparation (usually oral) they try.

Prescribing recommendations are given in subsequent chapters dealing with the use of HT for specific purposes.

1.3 For most women, the benefits of HT outweigh the risks

Many women are concerned about the side-effects associated with HT. These are described in more detail in Chapter 9. However, as with all medications, the potential advantages need to be weighed against the risks. For many women, the benefits of wisely prescribed HT far outweigh the risks. HT can reduce the acute symptoms of the climacteric and, in old age, postpone those insidious conditions that threaten the quality of life of both the elderly woman and her carers (Figure 1.2). There is little evidence that HT significantly increases life expectancy itself, but maintaining a good quality of life into old age and improving the health expectancy of women are valid goals of HT prescribing and research. These would allow women to retain their independence for longer, thus reducing their demands on national health and social services, and alleviating pressures on carers (Figure 1.1).

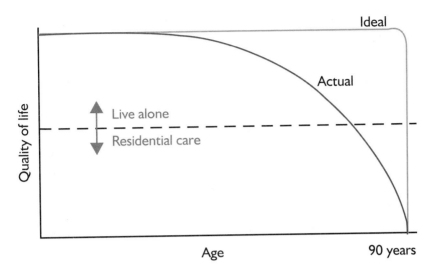

Figure 1.2

Graph showing ideal and actual quality of life with age. The use of hormone replacement therapy enables the 'actual' curve to be shifted to the right, towards the 'ideal'

References

1. Cooper C. Epidemiology of osteoporosis. *Osteoporos Int* 1999;9(Suppl 2):S2–8

2. National Statistics Online – Census 2001. http://www.statistics.gov.uk

3. *Pennell Report on Women's Health*. The Pennell Initiative, Health Services Management Unit, University of Manchester, 1998

4. Hobbs FB, Damon BL. 65+ in the United States. *Current Population Report P23-190*. Washington, DC: US Bureau of the Census, 1996

5.   World Bank Group. *PovertyNet*, 2000. Web address: http://www.worldbank.org/poverty

6.   Hope S, Rees MCP. Why do British women start and stop hormone replacement therapy. *J Br Menop Soc* 1995;1:26–7

7.   Randall S. Problems encountered by long-term hormone replacement therapy users. *Br J Fam Plann* 1990;16:101–5

Chapter 2

The principles of HT

2.1   HT has been used for over 70 years

In the eighteenth century, treatment of menopausal symptoms included the consumption of raw eggs and powdered penis of the ass, as well as the application of leeches to rid the body of toxins. One enlightened physician recommended: 'At meals she may be indulged with half a pint of old clear London porter or a glass of Rhenish wine'[1]. By the 1890s, the link between hot flushes and ovarian failure had been recognized. In Paris, women were prescribed sandwiches of sheep's ovaries in unleavened bread[2]! A few years later, ovarian extracts were administered by injection[3]. Estrogen itself was first used to treat menopausal symptoms in 1929 in the USA, and oral estrogen preparations became available in the late 1930s. The most widely used preparation, a mixture of estrogens extracted from the urine of pregnant mares, was available as early as 1943. Common terminology associated with HT is explained in Table 2.1 and the relationship between different time periods of the menopause are illustrated in Figure 2.1.

Table 2.1   Common terminology associated with the menopausal transition and climacteric. Adapted from Utian WH. The International Menopause Society menopause-related terminology definitions. *Climacteric* 1999;2:284–6

Term	Characteristics
Menopause (natural menopause)	the term natural menopause is defined as the permanent cessation of menstruation resulting from the loss of ovarian follicular activity. Natural menopause is recognized to have occurred after 12 consecutive months of amenorrhea, for which there is no other obvious pathological or physiological cause. Menopause occurs with the final menstrual period which is known with certainty only in retrospect a year or more after the event. An adequate independent biological marker for the event does not exist
Perimenopause	the term perimenopause should include the time immediately prior to the menopause (when the endocrinological, biological and clinical features of approaching menopause commence) and the first year after menopause
Menopausal transition	the term menopausal transition should be reserved for the time before the final menstrual period when variability in the menstrual cycle is usually increased. This term can be used synonymously with 'premenopause', although this latter term can be confusing and preferably should be abandoned
Climacteric	the phase in the aging of women marking the transition from the reproductive phase to the non-reproductive state. This phase incorporates the perimenopause, by extending for a longer variable period before and after the perimenopause
Climacteric syndrome	the climacteric is sometimes, but not necessarily always, associated with symptomatology. When this occurs, it may be termed the 'climacteric syndrome'
Premenopause	the term premenopause is often used ambiguously, either to refer to the 1 or 2 years immediately before the menopause or to refer to the whole of the reproductive period prior to the menopause. The group recommended that the term be used consistently in the latter sense to encompass the entire reproductive period up to the final menstrual period
Postmenopause	the term postmenopause is defined as dating from the final menstrual period, regardless of whether the menopause was induced or spontaneous

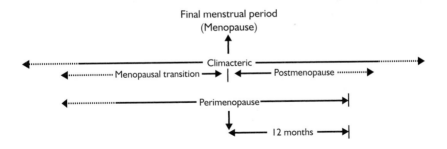

Figure 2.1

Illustration of the relationship between different time periods surrounding the menopause. Adapted from WHO Report 96238. Geneva: World Health Organization, 1994

2.2   Natural estrogens are used in HT

Estrogen is the collective name for a number of different, naturally occurring steroids with similar biological effects. The main human estrogens are estradiol (mainly from the ovary), estrone and estriol.

The estrogens most commonly used in HT, especially in North America, are the conjugated equine estrogens obtained from pregnant mares' urine. A mixture of these estrogens (mainly estrone) is used in an oral preparation, marketed as Premarin®. Some of the estrogens in Premarin are specific to horses, but they are chemically very similar to human hormones and have comparable, although not identical, effects. Most of the research into HT has been in women treated with this formulation[4] and it is possible that some of the observed clinical effects result from the different biological activities of the various constituents of the mixture. In the UK and Europe, pure estradiol, synthesized from soy beans and yams, is more widely prescribed. As this is identical to the naturally occurring hormone and avoids the issue of animal welfare, some women prefer it. Whether the results obtained

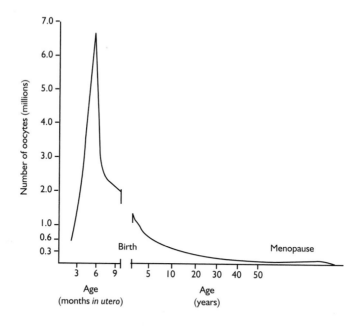

Figure 2.2

Changes in the number of oocytes from fetal life to menopause. Data from Baker TG. Oogenesis and ovulation. In Austin CR, Short RV, eds. *Reproduction in Mammals, Vol. 1. Germ Cells and Fertilization*. London: Cambridge University Press, 1972:14

from studies with Premarin can be extrapolated to pure estradiol is a matter of some debate, although a number of studies indicate that they have similar protective effects in terms of bone mass and the cardiovascular system[5–7].

2.3 Hormonal changes during the menopausal period provide the rationale for the use of HT

The female sex hormone, estradiol, is produced in the ovary by cells which develop in conjunction with the developing oocyte. The menopause occurs when the ovary runs out of oocytes (Figure 2.2), and so stops producing enough estradiol to support the menstrual cycle. The typical acute menopausal symptoms of hot flushes and sweats, disturbed sleep and lethargy and, later, dry vagina and some urinary problems, are caused by the decline in circulating levels of estrogen.

The menstrual cycle

The menstrual cycle is controlled by a complex process, involving hormones produced by the pituitary gland (gonadotropins), which stimulate production of the ovarian hormones, estrogen and progesterone. The fluctuations in the levels of the gonadotropins – follicle stimulating hormone (FSH) and luteinizing hormone (LH) – and of the ovarian hormones in relation to the developing follicle are shown in Figure 2.3.

In the premenopausal woman, in the first half of the menstrual cycle the release of estrogen stimulates the lining of the uterus (the endometrium), causing it to become thicker. After the mid-cycle release of a mature ovum, progesterone is produced by the ovarian cells. Progesterone inhibits the proliferation of the endometrium, causing it to develop secretory glandular tissue, which would nourish the embryo should implantation occur. In the absence of implantation, the levels of circulating progesterone decline and menstruation results. The cycle restarts and estrogen levels rise again.

Perimenopausal changes in hormone production

The number of oocytes present in the female is determined during fetal development, reaching a maximum between 20 and 28 weeks of gestation. From the time when a girl begins to have periods, there is a gradual reduction until, at about 50 years of age, the reserve of oocytes is depleted (Figure 2.2). In the years immediately preceding the menopause, the production of both estrogen and progesterone falls gradually, in tandem with the reduction in oocyte numbers. The pituitary gland augments its production of FSH and LH, in an attempt to force secretion of the ovarian hormones from an increasingly unresponsive ovary.

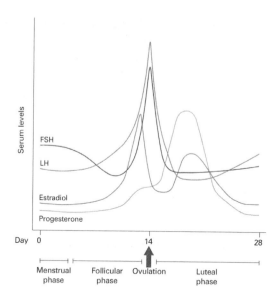

Figure 2.3

Serum levels of gonadotropins and ovarian hormones during the menstrual cycle (levels are not to scale). Luteinizing hormone (LH) stimulates androgen production in thecal cells of the developing follicle. At the same time, follicle stimulating hormone (FSH) induces estrogen production in the granulosa cells. Ovulation follows the LH surge at about day 14. During the luteal phase, both progesterone and estrogen are produced by the granulosa cells. In the absence of fertilization, declines in estrogen and progesterone levels lead to menstruation. Redrawn from Henderson VW. *Hormone Therapy and the Brain: A Clinical Perspective on the Role of Estrogen.* Carnforth, UK: Parthenon Publishing Group, 2000

At this stage, many cycles fail to release an ovum and this can result in heavier and less regular periods (Figure 2.4). The length of the menstrual cycle may alter (becoming either longer or shorter). Typical menopausal symptoms are experienced by about 80% of women at this time. Eventually, despite the increased production of pituitary hormones, there is insufficient circulating estrogen to stimulate growth of the endometrium. As a result, periods stop – the woman has reached her menopause. High circulating levels of FSH and LH are indicative of the menopausal

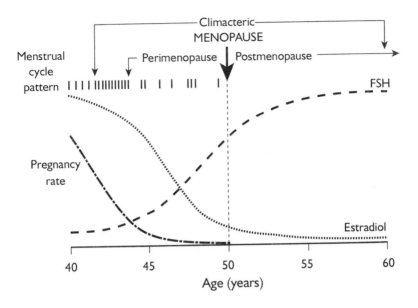

Figure 2.4

Changes in a woman's fifth and sixth decades of life. The menopause is marked by the last physiological period and is preceded by the menstrual cycle irregularity of the perimenopause. The beginning of the menopause transition is called the climacteric. FSH, follicle stimulating hormone. Redrawn from Soules MR, Battaglia DE, Klein NA. The endocrinology of ovarian (reproductive) aging in women. In Te Velde ER, Pearson PL, Broekmans FJ, eds. *Female Reproductive Aging*. Carnforth, UK: Parthenon Publishing, 2000

state, and can be measured by a simple blood test. This is not usually necessary in women whose periods have ceased after the age of 45 years, but can be useful in younger women who are experiencing infrequent or absent periods, to test whether this is due to premature ovarian failure.

Estrogen-only replacement therapies and the risk of endometrial cancer

The estrogen component of HT replaces the estrogen lost at the menopause and reduces or eliminates typical menopausal symptoms. However, its action on the endometrium is similar to that of the endogenous hormone, which is to trigger endometrial thickening. In the absence of ovulation, the menopausal woman does not produce enough progesterone to limit endometrial growth. Thus, the endometrium is not shed, and the woman does not bleed. This continuous stimulation of the endometrium by estrogen, unopposed by progesterone, may cause hyperplasia (abnormal thickening of the uterine lining). Although this is not necessarily harmful, in a small number of cases it can progress to atypical changes in the glandular cells, which have a greater potential than normal cells to progress to endometrial cancer. Grady and colleagues[8] analyzed the results of 30 studies carried out between 1970 and 1994, and calculated that the risk of endometrial cancer was increased by a factor of 2.3 when estrogen alone (i.e. *unopposed* estrogen) was used for up to 5 years. The risk was increased approximately ten-fold when the treatment was extended to over 10 years. Furthermore, the elevated risk continued for several years after treatment was stopped. Endometrial cancer is a rare condition with a varying prevalence around the world. In the WHI study of North American women with a mean age of 63 years the incidence was 2 per 10 000 per year. With unopposed estrogen this could, therefore, increase to 2 per 1000 per year with long-term use. While this remains a low level of risk, it has widely been considered unacceptable, and that women with an intact uterus should always be prescribed HT with a progesterone-like component. However, this view has now been questioned following the Million Women Study (MWS) report showing that combined therapy (sequential or continuous combined) is associated with a four times greater risk of breast cancer than unopposed estrogen, so the balance of risks needs careful consideration[9].

2.4 Including a progestogen in HT reduces the risk of endometrial cancer

Progesterone in its naturally occurring form is not suitable for use to protect the endometrium, as it is metabolized rapidly in the gut and liver when taken by mouth. The high dose of oral

Table 2.2   Daily doses of progestogen needed for endometrial protection

	Oral	Transdermal
Sequential		
Norethisterone	0.7–1 mg for last 10–14 days of 28-day cycle	170 or 250 µg for last 14 days of 28-day cycle
Levonorgestrel	75–250 µg for last 10-14 days of 28-day cycle	20 µg for last 14 days of 28-day cycle
Medroxyprogesterone acetate	5–10 mg for the last 14 days of 28-day cycle	
	20 mg for the last 14 days of 3-month cycle	
Dydrogesterone	10–20 mg for the last 14 days of 28-day cycle	
Continuous combined		
Norethisterone	0.5–1 mg	170 µg
Medroxyprogesterone acetate	2.5–5 mg	
Dydrogesterone	5 mg	

progesterone that is necessary to attain therapeutic blood levels produces unwanted sedative side-effects. There is a formulation available for rectal use, but to date there is little information available regarding effectiveness in protecting the endometrium. Natural progesterone creams do not safeguard the endometrium, as therapeutic blood levels are not achieved and the endometrium remains proliferative. Thus, these creams are not suitable for use as the progesterone component of HT[10].

Several synthetic progesterone-like compounds (progestogens) have been developed, which are not subject to the rapid metabolic degradation seen with progesterone (Table 2.2). Their role in HT is to protect the endometrium and reduce hyperplasia[11]. Progestogens can be given *sequentially* with estrogen, for 10–14 days in the second half of the cycle, and bleeding usually occurs towards the end of this phase or when the progestogen is withdrawn (Table 2.2). This mimics the natural course of events in the normal menstrual cycle. Given at an adequate dosage (Table 2.2) for at least 12 days, progestogen reduces the incidence of hyperplasia to almost 0% with short-term use.

Sequential treatment can be continued for up to 5 years with no increase in risk of endometrial cancer. However, recent research[12] has demonstrated that, in postmenopausal women, the protective effect of progesterone is reduced after 5 years of sequential therapy. The current thinking is to change from sequential to continuous combined therapy (Table 2.2) in women who are at least 1 year postmenopausal. When administered in a continuous regimen, progestogens inhibit the effects of estrogen, so that in most cases the endometrium does not proliferate and remains atrophic. UK research[13] has shown that continuous combined therapy can also reverse existing hyperplasia and that this is more protective against endometrial cancer than no treatment. After 5 years of the continuous combined regimen, the endometrium remains normal[14]. This has the added advantage of being a period-free treatment (although it may take several months for bleeding to stop completely). Lower doses of progestogen can be used, and this, along with the effect of a constant, rather than cyclical, hormonal milieu, reduces side-effects.

2.5 How and when to change from sequential to continuous combined therapy

Most women do not like the bleed associated with sequential HT and would prefer to switch to a period-free regimen as soon as possible. When HT is started before the menopause there is no way of determining when the last period would have occurred. Breakthrough bleeding while taking continuous combined HT is most common during the early months, especially if there is still some ovarian activity. A statistical guideline is that by the age of 54 years, 80% of women will be at least 1 year postmenopause.

The changeover to the continuous combined regimen should take place after the bleed at the end of a cycle of sequential therapy.

2.6　Tibolone – an alternative to continuous combined HT

Tibolone is a synthetic steroid that is related to testosterone, the male hormone, but it has some estrogen-, progesterone- and testosterone-like effects. It has been extensively researched and is licensed for the relief of menopausal symptoms, including reduced libido, and for the prevention of postmenopausal osteo-porosis. Its mode of action has been described as 'tissue specific' as it has different effects in different tissues. In the endometrium it has a potent progesterone effect, producing a thin and atrophic lining. However, breast density, as measured by mammography, is less affected than by continuous combined HT. To date, long-term benefits and risks have not been fully assessed. (As tibolone cannot strictly be classed as HT and it is not a selective estrogen receptor modulator (SERM), Professor David Purdie has suggested a new acronym, SPEAR, selective progesterone, estrogen and androgen regulator[15].)

2.7　Hormones are being developed which will provide the long-term advantages of estrogen without the disadvantages

Estrogen is, by far, the most effective treatment currently available for the alleviation of acute menopausal symptoms, such as hot flushes and urogenital complaints. In the longer term, it is the therapy of choice for many women to prevent the loss of bone mass and thus avoid osteoporosis. It may reduce the risk of cardiovascular disease, and evidence is accumulating that it may delay the onset of Alzheimer's disease. Recent evidence has confirmed a reduction in colorectal cancer associated with HT use[16]. Against this must be set a small increase in the risk of breast cancer and its effects on the endometrium, with the attendant drawbacks of progestogen use and breakthrough bleeding (Chapter 8). The ideal therapy for long-term use would be 'bone good, bleed-free and breast safe'[17]. Such a therapy is becoming a reality with the development of the so-called 'designer hormones', the Selective Estrogen Receptor Modulators, or SERMs.

Estrogen acts within the cell by combining with a receptor molecule (Figure 2.5). The resulting estrogen–receptor complex then binds to specific sites in the DNA, triggering a series of reactions, which leads to the manufacture of new proteins. These, in turn, affect the metabolism of target cells in the reproductive system, the breasts, the cardiovascular system, the brain and central nervous system, the skeleton, skin and connective tissues.

The 1980s saw the development of a number of antiestrogens, which were designed to block the action of estrogen on receptors in estrogen-sensitive breast cells. The best known of these is tamoxifen. In the early 1990s, Love and colleagues discovered that postmenopausal women with breast cancer, who were treated with tamoxifen, had lower serum cholesterol levels and greater spinal bone density than untreated controls[18, 19].

The results of these studies indicated that tamoxifen imitates the effects of estrogen in the liver and in bone, whilst blocking its effect in the breast. More recent research has discovered the existence of several distinct estrogen receptors, concentrated in different tissues, which initiate manifold chemical responses in cells. Drugs such as tamoxifen react selectively with these different receptors to regulate (modulate) their activity, hence the name, SERMS.

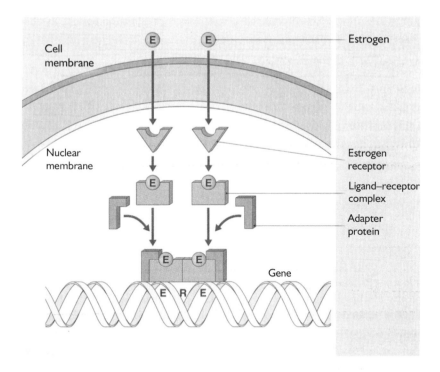

Figure 2.5

Transcriptional regulation by estrogen. Binding of estrogen (E) to its receptor occurs in the cell nucleus, leading to a dissociation of complexed proteins and a conformational change in the receptor shape. Two ligand–receptor complexes join to form a dimer, which in association with adaptor proteins, attaches to the estrogen response element (ERE) site on the genome, resulting in transcriptional regulation of a downstream gene. Reproduced from Henderson VW. *Hormone Therapy and the Brain: A Clinical Perspective on the Role of Estrogen*. Carnforth, UK: Parthenon Publishing, 2000

While tamoxifen has been proven to have excellent estrogen-blocking effects in the breast, and to offer some protection to the cardiovascular system and skeleton, it mimics the action of estrogen on the endometrium, causing an increased risk of irregular bleeding, endometrial polyps, hyperplasia and cancer. For this reason, it is not an ideal long-term alternative to HT.

In controlled trials, another SERM, called raloxifene, increased bone density, produced a favorable alteration in blood lipid levels and, most significantly, reduced the risk of breast cancer[20]. The side-effects were similar in both the treatment and control groups, with the exception of mild to moderate hot flushes, which were greater for the first 6 months in the treatment group. Crucially, raloxifene does not stimulate the endometrium, making it a promising choice for the treatment of osteoporosis in older menopausal women. It is licensed in the UK and the USA for the treatment of osteoporosis, and further trials are underway to assess its suitability for use with breast cancer patients.

References

1. Leeke J. *Chronic or Slow Diseases Peculiar to Women*. London: Baldwin, 1777

2. Richardson RG. *The Menopause – A Neglected Crisis*. Queenborough: Abbott Laboratories, 1973

3. Novak E. The management of the menopause. *Am J Obstet Gynecol* 1940;40:585–9

4. Lobo RA. Benefits and risks of estrogen replacement therapy. *Am J Obstet Gynecol* 1995;173(Suppl 3):982–9

5. Hillard TC, Whitcroft SJ, Marsh MS, *et al.* Long-term effects of transdermal and oral hormone replacement therapy on post-menopausal bone loss. *Osteoporos Int* 1994;4:341–8

6. Grodstein F, Stampfer MJ. The epidemiology of coronary heart disease and estrogen replacement therapy in postmenopausal women. *Prog Cardiovasc Dis* 1995;3:199–210

7. Falkeborn M, Persson I, Adami HO, *et al.* The risk of acute myocardial infarction after estrogen and estrogen–progestogen replacement. *Br J Obstet Gynaecol* 1992;99:821–8

8. Grady D, Gebretsadik T, Marsh MS, *et al.* Hormone replacement therapy and endometrial cancer risk: a meta-analysis. *Obstet Gynecol* 1995;85:304–13

9. Million Women Study Collaborators. Breast cancer and hormone replacement in the Million Women Study. *Lancet* 2003;362:419–27

10. Wren BG, McFarland K, Edwards L, *et al.* Effect of sequential transdermal progesterone cream on endometrium, bleeding pattern, and plasma progesterone and salivary progesterone levels in postmenopausal women. *Climacteric* 2000;3:155–60

11. The Writing Group of the PEPI Trial. Effects of hormone replacement therapy on endometrial histology in post-menopausal women. The postmenopausal estrogen/progestin interventions (PEPI) trial. *J Am Med Assoc* 1996;275:370–5

12. Beresford SAA, Weiss NS, Voigt LF, McKnight B. Risk of endometrial cancer in relation to the use of estrogen combined with cyclic progestogen therapy in postmenopausal women. *Lancet* 1997;349:458–61

13. Sturdee DW, Ulrich LG, Barlow DH, *et al.* The endometrial response to sequential and continuous combined estrogen–progestogen replacement therapy. *Br J Obstet Gynaecol* 2000;107:1392–400

14. Wells M, Sturdee DW, Barlow DH, *et al*. Effect on endometrium of long term treatment with continuous combined oestrogen–progestogen replacement therapy: a follow-up study. *Br Med J* 2002;325:239–42

15. Purdie DW. What is tibolone – and is it a SPEAR? *Climacteric* 2002;5:236–9

16. Writing Group for the Women's Health Initiative Investigators. Risks and benefits of estrogen plus progestin in healthy post-menopausal women. *J Am Med Assoc* 2002;288:321–33

17. Purdie DW. Potential applications of SERMS. In *SERMS, A New Choice for Postmenopausal Health. Proceedings of a Satellite Symposium at the Sixth Bath Conference on Osteoporosis*, 1998:10–12

18. Love RR, Mazess RB, Barden HS, *et al*. Effects of tamoxifen on bone mineral density in postmenopausal women with breast cancer. *N Engl J Med* 1992;326:852–6

19. Love RR, Newcomb PA, Wiebe DA, *et al*. Effects of tamoxifen therapy on lipid and lipoprotein levels in postmenopausal patients with node-negative breast cancer. *J Natl Cancer Inst* 1990;82:1327–32

20. Cauley JA, Norton L, Lippman ME, *et al*. Continued breast cancer risk reduction in postmenopausal women treated with raloxifene: 4-year results from the MORE trial. *Breast Cancer Treat* 2001;65:125–34

Chapter 3

HT delivery routes and regimens

3.1 Oral preparations of HT are the most commonly used, but are not suitable for all women

In the absence of contraindications, the oral route is usually the first choice of treatment (Table 3.1). It is simple to use, and cheaper than other delivery routes. Both conjugated equine estrogens and estradiol are effective in relieving acute menopausal symptoms and are well tolerated by most women,

Table 3.1   Advantages and disadvantages of oral estrogen therapy

Advantages	Disadvantages
Easy to take	High dose required
Cheap	Variation in absorption
Good control	Alters liver protein synthesis
Short half-life	Minor side-effects
Wide choice	Daily dosage
	All tablets contain lactose

although nausea and other minor side-effects are more likely with the oral route. In the long term, oral preparations provide effective protection for the cardiovascular system and the skeleton.

Oral estrogen preparations are absorbed through the gut, before being carried directly to the liver in the hepatic portal system. The liver converts the estradiol to estrone[1] and it is in this form that most of the estrogen enters the general circulation. This has two important effects. First, up to 90% of the administered dose is inactivated, so higher doses of estrogens have to be given to reach therapeutic plasma levels. This also results in inconsistent blood levels between patients. Second, the estrogen stimulates the liver to produce triglycerides (a type of fat) and plasma levels of triglycerides rise. Elevated levels of plasma triglycerides have been implicated in cardiovascular disease and it is advisable for women with raised triglyceride levels to avoid oral estrogen therapy. In contrast, transdermal patches reduce triglyceride levels by 15–20%[2] (see Section 6.6). Oral estrogen reduces insulin resistance, which is less affected by transdermal estrogen.

In the premenopausal woman, the ratio of estradiol to estrone in the plasma is about 2:1. In the postmenopausal woman, total estrogen is reduced, although some estrone is produced in adipose (fat) tissue so the estradiol:estrone ratio is reversed, and becomes 1:2. The production of estrone is proportional to the amount of adipose tissue; therefore, women who are overweight have fewer symptoms but also a greater risk of estrogen-related tumors, which may lead to breast or endometrial cancer.

It is a matter of debate whether an aim of giving HT should be to restore the estradiol:estrone ratio to that typical of the premenopausal woman. This cannot be achieved with oral estrogens, which are metabolized in the liver and intestine.

For a small number of women with lactose intolerance, oral administration of estrogen is not an appropriate treatment as all the preparations contain lactose as a bulking agent for the tablet.

However, lactose is not a constituent of estrogen preparations given by other routes.

3.2 Transdermal systems – an acceptable alternative to the oral route

Estrogen is absorbed easily through the skin, vaginal epithelium, and the lining of the nose. Breakdown in the gut and liver is avoided, so a lower dose can be used and higher estradiol levels are achieved in the systemic circulation. The estradiol : estrone ratio is closer to that of the premenopausal woman. While there is no evidence that this is necessary, it could be argued that it is more physiologically 'normal' and, therefore, more desirable. The transdermal route also avoids the gastric side-effects sometimes seen with oral preparations.

Patches

Transdermal patches are attached to the skin below the waist. With the early alcohol-containing patches, skin irritation was a problem in about one-third of women, but recently developed systems, which use a thin matrix, largely avoid this. Most patches have to be changed twice weekly, but some can remain *in situ* for up to 7 days. A number of patches containing progestogen have now been developed for sequential therapy, and two for continuous combined therapy.

Gels

A gel containing estradiol has been the most popular method of administration of HT in France for the past 20 years. It is dispensed from a non-pressurized cannister, and is licensed in the UK for the relief of menopausal symptoms and osteoporosis prevention. A similar gel is available in a sachet. Measured doses of gel are rubbed into the skin of the arms or legs, absorption is rapid, and symptomatic relief is comparable to that of orally and patch-administered estradiol.

The gel is invisible once rubbed into the skin and bathing or swimming are possible.

Nasal spray

Estrogen is absorbed easily through the nasal mucosa, which has a rich blood supply and a surface area of about 160 cm². This novel route has similar advantages to transdermal systems, with the avoidance of intestinal and liver metabolism[3]. An intranasal estradiol spray has been developed and licensed. Daily administration of the spray provides a pulse of estrogen, which reaches its peak value in the blood within 10–30 minutes and returns to pretreatment levels within 12 hours, which is very different to the more sustained levels of hormones observed with oral or patch administration (Figure 3.1). However, symptom relief is as good as that achieved with other routes and there may be fewer side-effects. The effects on bone mass and other tissues

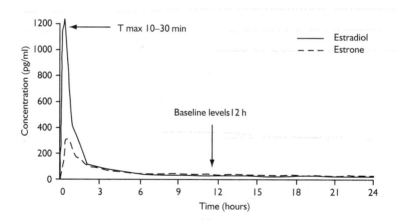

Figure 3.1

Pharmacokinetic profile following a single dose of Aerodiol 300 µg nasal spray. (Conversion factor: pg/nl x 3.67 = pmol/l). Data from Devissaguet J-Ph, Brian N, Lhote O, *et al.* Pulsed estrogen therapy: pharmacokinetics of intranasal 17-β-estradiol (S21400) in postmenopausal women and comparison with oral and transdermal formulations. *Eur J Drug Metab Pharmacokinet* 1999;24:265–71

also appear to be comparable. These findings suggest that blood levels of estrogen are not necessarily indicative of what is happening in the tissues.

Vaginal formulations

Menopausal symptoms sometimes include vaginal dryness, which can cause pain or discomfort during intercourse, as well as urinary infections and incontinence. These symptoms are not always alleviated immediately by systemic treatment, and additional local treatment may be needed to 'prime' the urogenital tissues. For the older woman who wants to relieve her urogenital symptoms but does not want systemic treatment, local vaginal preparations may be appropriate[4] (see Section 4.6 and Appendix for list of preparations).

Very little estrogen reaches the general circulation from these preparations and there are no effects on other menopausal symptoms if the recommended doses are used. However, a recently developed vaginal ring releases sufficient estrogen to relieve menopausal symptoms and to have local benefits on the vagina and bladder. These benefits last for up to 3 months. It is a discreet and effective method of administration without adverse effects on sexual enjoyment for either partner.

Implants

Estrogen implants have been available for more than 50 years, and for most of this time they were the only alternative to oral therapy. The implants contain 25 or 50 mg of crystalloid estradiol and are inserted under the skin with the aid of a local anesthetic and special introducer. Once in place, the implants slowly release the active hormone into the subcutaneous fatty tissue, from where they reach the circulation. Renewal is necessary at about 6-monthly intervals.

Implants are particularly suitable and convenient for women after hysterectomy who do not need to take progestogen, as once inserted they can be forgotten until reimplantation is due. For the woman with an intact uterus, this is a marginal benefit as she still has to remember to use progestogen, either orally, transdermally or intrauterine (see Section 3.3).

Good symptomatic relief and bone mass protection are achieved with implants, which may be better than with oral therapy. However, each pellet may continue to release estradiol for 2 years or more, and this can lead to blood levels well above normal if implants are given too frequently. It is not known if this is clinically hazardous, but it is inadvisable and, theoretically at least, there is an increased risk of complications such as breast cancer. In recent years there has been much concern about tachyphylaxis. This is the term used for the situation in which a woman requests repeated implants because she is experiencing a return of symptoms at increasingly shorter intervals. However, these symptoms are not usually typical of estrogen deficiency, and many such women have some degree of psychopathology[5]. This situation can be avoided by giving implants at intervals of no less than 6 months and at dosages of no more than 25–50 mg at a time. In addition, regular blood tests should be carried out to check whether the estradiol level exceeds the normal range (about 300–1000 pmol/l).

Non-biodegradable estradiol implants are currently under development. These are intended to give a more constant level of estradiol in the circulation and could last for 1–2 years.

Testosterone implants

This hormone also can be given by implant for women who have an unsatisfactory response to estrogen alone. This is especially the case if they are troubled by loss of energy, headaches, depression and, particularly, loss of libido[6]. Testosterone is usually administered at the same time as estradiol, but can be given as a supplement to other routes of administration. However, androgenic side-effects may occur, such as an increase in downy facial hair or mild voice changes.

Transdermal patches are currently being evaluated as an alternative route of administration of testosterone. The oral route is not suitable because of the adverse effects resulting from high levels of the hormone passing directly from the intestines to the liver.

Injections of testosterone are available for men with androgen deficiency who need a much higher dose, but these have to be given every month and this is not a licensed method of administration for postmenopausal women.

3.3   The progestogen-releasing intrauterine device – a new development in HT

The levonorgestrel-containing intrauterine system (IUS), known as Mirena® (Figure 3.2), is licensed in the UK for contraception and for the treatment of heavy periods. It releases low-dose progestogen (20 µg levonorgestrel/day) directly into the uterine cavity, where it causes atrophy of the endometrium, which tends

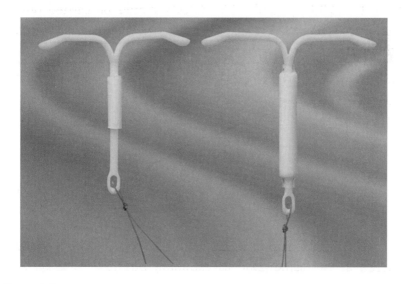

Figure 3.2

The levonorgestrel-releasing intrauterine device, Mirena®. The version on the left is smaller, designed for the older woman

to stop periods completely. It is appropriate to emphasize that, in the menopausal woman, progestogen is required only to protect the endometrium – it is not necessary elsewhere in the body. Furthermore, there is no need to have a regular bleed, as the uterus can remain perfectly healthy without it. The protective effect of progestogen arises, not because of withdrawal bleeding, but because it inhibits the stimulatory effects of estrogen on the cells of the endometrium. It makes sense, therefore, to localize the progestogen at the site of action and to minimize the dose that reaches the general circulation. In this respect, the IUS is ideal. This system can double up as a contraceptive for perimenopausal women and, together with oral or transdermal estrogen, can provide an alternative method of continuous combined therapy[7]. It is also valuable for women who suffer from irregular uterine bleeding prior to the menopause, caused by the run-down of the control system of the menstrual cycle. If bleeding continues despite attempts to control it with the other formulations available, this IUS can be the best option and avoids the need to consider more extensive alternatives, such as hysterectomy.

A smaller version for use with older postmenopausal women (who have a smaller uterus) is in the process of development, although it will be several years before it becomes available[8]. Once inserted, the low dose of progestogen that is released into the bloodstream causes few side-effects and the device can remain *in situ* for up to 5 years.

3.4 Women at different stages of the menopausal process benefit from different HT regimens (Table 3.2; Figure 3.3)

Sequential regimens

For women who have not had a hysterectomy and are in the perimenopausal stage, the sequential regimen is the most suitable. Continuous estrogen is taken along with progestogen for 10–14

Table 3.2   HT regimens

Regimen	Details	Comments
Sequential	estrogen daily, progestogen for last 10–14 days of cycle	withdrawal bleeding every month; change to CCEPT after 5 years (see Section 3.4)
Cyclical	estrogen on days 1–21, progestogen on days 9–21, nothing on days 22–28	withdrawal bleeding every month; change to CCEPT after 5 years
Long-cycle	estrogen for 3 months, progestogen in second half of third month	withdrawal bleeding every third month; long-term protection of endometrium uncertain; suitable for short-term use during transition, before changing to CCEPT
Continuous combined	estrogen and progestogen continuously	in theory, no bleeding should occur, and the endometrium should remain atrophic, but many women experience irregular bleeding for the first few months (nearly always settles down); suitable only for women aged over 54 or who are at least 1 year postmenopause (prior to this there is still some ovarian activity and break through bleeding may occur); if the woman was using CCEPT this would have to be investigated to exclude endometrial abnormality; compliance is usually better than with regimens which induce bleeding
Tibolone	synthetic derivative of testosterone, given continuously	has weak estrogenic, androgenic and progestogenic properties; does not stimulate uterine lining, can be used without progestogen and causes less breakthrough bleeding than other regimens; relieves menopausal symptoms, including bone loss; may not provide the same protection against cardiovascular disease because of its relatively weak estrogenic effects; suitable only for women aged over 54 or who have had no periods for at least 12 months

CCEPT, continuous combined estrogen and progestogen therapy

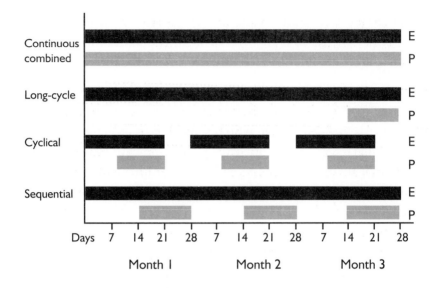

Figure 3.3

Hormone therapy regimens showing the days of each cycle on which estrogen (E; black bars) or progestogen (P; grey bars) are taken

days in the second half of the menstrual cycle. Bleeding occurs when the progestogen is stopped, although it often starts before the end of the progestogen phase. Progestogen can be given orally, transdermally, by vaginal gel or IUS. Some cyclic regimens have 21 days of hormone followed by a 7-day tablet-free stage, but there is no evidence that this is advantageous and some women experience a return of symptoms during the tablet-free week. This regimen also seems illogical as the ovary does not stop producing estrogen for 7 days during the normal menstrual cycle.

In pre- or perimenopausal women who are still menstruating, it is important to attempt to synchronize the HT cycle with the natural cycle, to avoid additional bleeds.

Sequential therapy can also be used for postmenopausal women. However, the withdrawal bleed is a problem, especially for those women several years past the menopause who have become accustomed to a period-free existence, and it is a major reason for non-compliance with treatment. There are two options – long-cycle therapy for women just past the menopause and continuous combined therapies or tibolone for older women (see below).

As progestogen is required for endometrial protection only, women who have had a hysterectomy can be given continuous estrogen alone. A woman who has had her ovaries removed faces additional years without the protection of estrogen, with potential adverse consequences for her cardiovascular system and skeleton. Even when one or both ovaries are conserved at hysterectomy, there is a good chance that they will cease to function up to 4 years earlier than would have happened without the operation[9]. The former should use estrogen replacement therapy following her hysterectomy, and the latter should be monitored for signs of early ovarian failure and offered appropriate treatment.

Long-cycle therapy

This has similarities to monthly sequential therapy but has a progestogen phase every 3 months only, instead of every month. Withdrawal bleeding therefore occurs only four times a year and lasts an average of 5–6 days. Three months may be the longest cycle that can be used safely, since endometrial hyperplasia has been observed after 4 months of estrogen alone[10]. There is a higher incidence of breakthrough bleeding with long-cycle than with sequential therapy. Nevertheless, in one study, 80% of women who had previously used monthly sequential therapy favored the long-cycle regimen[11].

Continuous combined regimens

As its name suggests, continuous combined HT (CCEPT) involves taking both steroids at all times. There is no stage at which estrogen is taken alone, unlike in sequential therapy, and a combination of delivery routes can be used. The doses of continuous progestogen needed are at the lower end of the range for endometrial protection and this may help to minimize side-effects. The progestogen inhibits the proliferative effect of estrogen and the endometrium remains atrophic. Although this regimen is sometimes promoted as a 'no-bleed' treatment, in practice, up to 80% of women experience irregular bleeding for as long as 12 weeks after the start of the treatment. This is more common in women who are within 1 year of the menopause than in postmenopausal women. Frequently, only spotting is involved, and bleeding is uncommon after 12 months of use. For many older women this is a significant advantage.

Continuous combined treatment is not usually used for perimenopausal women, whose residual ovarian activity may cause an unacceptably high incidence of breakthrough bleeding. Although there is no medical risk from this, women find it unpredictable and messy, and usually prefer sequential treatment with its regular bleed. Thus, CCEPT is best reserved for women who are known to be at least 1 year past their menopause.

The issue of breakthrough bleeding is complex and poorly understood. Some women, who are well past the menopause and not on HT, experience occasional bleeding and, on investigation, are found to have a healthy uterus. Why they should bleed from an atrophic endometrium is not clear. The options for such women are to try a reduced dose or a different estrogen/progestogen combination. Again, the IUS may prove to be a suitable choice, although it is not yet licensed for such a situation.

A similar situation is sometimes found with women on CCEPT who have attained a period-free state, but who from time to time experience breakthrough bleeding. This may be connected with growth factors and the effect of progestogen on the blood supply to the endometrium. What is certain, however, is that progestogen is protective[12], and that for long-term use (more than 5 years), the continuous administration of progestogen in period-free regimens is more protective than sequential use[13]. Data from Sweden[14] and the USA[15] have also shown that for up to 5 years' use, the standard monthly sequential regimens of estrogen and progestogen are not associated with an increased risk of endometrial cancer. However, with longer-term use (more than 5 years), this protection may be gradually lost, whereas regimens in which progestogen is taken daily may even reduce the risk of uterine cancer compared with women not taking HT[14].

Tibolone

Another option for continuous therapy is the synthetic compound tibolone, which has effects similar to those of the sex hormones. It has been shown to be bone-protective but its effects on the cardiovascular system are, as yet, unknown. It is converted in the endometrium to a metabolite which has no estrogenic activity and which therefore does not stimulate growth. Breakthrough bleeding with tibolone has been reported to occur in 12% of women during 2 years of treatment[16].

References

1. Longcope C, Gorbach S, Goldin B, et al., The metabolism of estradiol: oral compared to intravenous administration. *J Steroid Biochem* 1985;23:1065–70

2. Bush TL, Miller VT. Effects of pharmacologic agents used during menopause: impact on lipids and lipoproteins. In Mishell D, ed. *Menopause: Physiology and Pharmacology.* Chigaco: Year Book Medical Publishers, 1986:187–208

3. Studd JWW, Pornel B, Marton I, et al., for the Aerodiol Study Group. Efficacy and acceptability of intranasal 17β-estradiol for menopausal symptoms: randomised dose response study. *Lancet* 1999;353:1574–8

4. Mettler L, Olsen PG. Long-term treatment of atrophic vaginitis with low dose estradiol vaginal tablets. *Maturitas* 1991;14:23–31

5. Pearce J, Horton K, Blake F, *et al*. Psychological effect of continuation versus discontinuation of HT by estrogen implants; a placebo controlled study. *J Psychosom Res* 1997;42:177–86

6. Brincat M, Magos A, Studd JWW. Subcutaneous hormone implants for the control of climacteric symptoms; a prospective study. *Lancet* 1984;1:16–18

7. Riphagen FR. Intrauterine application of progestins in hormone replacement therapy: a review. *Climacteric* 2000;3:199–212

8. Randaskoski T, Tapanainen J, Tomas E, *et al*. Intrauterine 10 µg and 20 µg levonorgestrel systems in postmenopausal women receiving oral oestrogen replacement therapy: clinical, endometrial and metabolic response. *Br J Obstet Gynaecol* 2002;109:136–44

9. Siddle N, Sarrel P, Whitehead M. The effect of hysterectomy on the age of ovarian failure: identification of a sub-group of women with premature loss of ovarian function and literature review. *Fertil Steril* 1987;47:94–100

10. Hirvonen E, Salmi J, Puolakka J, *et al*. Can progestin be limited to every third month only in postmenopausal women taking estrogen? *Maturitas* 1995;21:39–44

11. Ettinger B, Selby J, Citron JT, *et al*. Cyclic hormone replacement therapy using quarterly progestin. *Obstet Gynecol* 1994; 83:693–700

12. The Writing Group of the PEPI Trial. Effects of hormone replacement therapy on endometrial histology in postmenopausal women. The postmenopausal estrogen/progestin interventions (PEPI) trial. *J Am Med Assoc* 1996;275:370–5

13. Wells M, Sturdee DW, Barlow DH, *et al.* Effect on endometrium of long-term treatment with continuous combined oestrogen–progestogen replacement therapy: a follow-up study. *Br Med J* 2002;325:239–42

14. Weiderpass E, Adami HO, Barron JA, *et al.* Risk of endometrial cancer following estrogen replacement with and without progestins. *J Natl Cancer Inst* 1999;91:1131–7

15. Beresford SAA, Weiss NS, Voigt LF, McKnight B. Risk of endometrial cancer in relation to use of estrogen combined with cyclic progestogen therapy in postmenopausal women. *Lancet* 1997;349:458–61

16. Völker W, Coelingh Bennink HJT, Helmond FA. Effects of tibolone on the endometrium. *Climacteric* 2001;4:203–8

Chapter 4

The control of climacteric symptoms

4.1 Maintaining quality of life in the climacteric

A list of typical acute menopausal symptoms makes for depressing reading (Table 4.1), and it is easy to form the impression that this is a stressful and debilitating time for most women. Yet many women report that their experience of the menopause is much less fraught than they had anticipated[1].

Table 4.1 Typical physical symptoms of the menopause

Acute physical symptoms of the climacteric	Medium-term physical symptoms of the postmenopause
Hot flushes	Vaginal dryness
Sweats	Pain or discomfort during intercourse
Night sweats	Urinary infections
Disturbed sleep	Pain on voiding
Lethargy	'Overactive' bladder (urge incontinence)
	Loss of skin elasticity

Studies in several countries have confirmed that, for many women, a natural menopause gives rise to few negative experiences. Hot flushes were the main symptom and little psychological distress was reported[2].

There is also evidence that experiences of the menopause are partly determined by culture. For example, it is known that Japanese women experience fewer menopausal symptoms than women in the West, and this is often attributed to their high consumption of phytoestrogens (plant estrogens), derived from soy products. Studies in India, Africa and some Arab countries reported few menopausal symptoms other than menstrual cycle changes. It is possible that, in cultures where older people are valued for their experience and wisdom, women welcome the menopause. Or perhaps there are social taboos against talking about the menopause and the distress is kept hidden.

There is undoubtedly a proportion of women whose symptoms are sufficiently unpleasant for them to seek help. The typical acute menopausal symptoms of hot flushes and sweats, known as vasomotor symptoms, are most marked during the transition years just before and after the menopause[3]. Figure 4.1 shows the average ages of the onset of various physical changes that may occur during the climacteric. These symptoms are often worst in women who have lost their ovaries to surgery or radiotherapy, because they experience a sudden drop in estrogen compared with the gradual decline of the normal menopause. Some women also suffer from breast tenderness, nausea and migraine. Such early symptoms typically last for 2 years, but can go on for up to 5 years[4]. For a few unfortunate women, these symptoms can continue indefinitely unless treated.

Some 5–8 years following the menopause, other menopausal symptoms occur with greater frequency. These are problems of the vagina and urinary tract, including vaginal dryness, pain on intercourse, urinary and vaginal infections and urinary urgency.

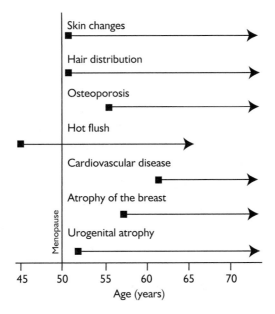

Figure 4.1

Average ages of the onset of physical changes that may occur during the climacteric

Psychological disturbances, such as depressed mood, tiredness, reduced sex drive, loss of confidence, and poor memory and concentration, are common complaints of women attending menopause clinics. Aging is naturally associated with these and various physical changes and the distinction between the effects of estrogen loss and those due to age is not always clear. The effect of the menopause and HT on psychological factors and mood is covered in Chapter 7.

4.2   HT is not necessary for every menopausal woman

HT is not a panacea for all the problems associated with middle and later life. Healthy women whose menopausal symptoms cause them little or no distress, and who have no obvious risk factors for cardiovascular disease, osteoporosis or Alzheimer's disease, will gain no major benefit from HT at the climacteric, and there is no need for them to take it. The early symptoms of hot flushes and sweats may not last long, and may be infrequent, so the value of HT is questionable in such cases. If symptoms such as atrophy (wasting) of the urogenital tract appear later, HT can be started then. The women who derive the greatest benefit from HT are those with severe symptoms which cause them distress.

4.3   HT alleviates vasomotor symptoms

Since these menopausal symptoms result from the reduction of endogenous estrogens, it follows that estrogen replacement will alleviate them. This has been known for over 40 years and is backed up by a considerable body of evidence[5-8].

Vasomotor symptoms

Hot flushes are disagreeable sensations of heat, which start in the face, head, neck or chest and spread across the body to a greater or lesser extent (Figure 4.2). They are often accompanied by a red face, sweating or dizziness, and can last from a few minutes to an hour. Some women experience them irregularly, whereas others may have them several times per hour. They can be triggered by spicy food, caffeine, alcohol and changes in temperature. Hot flushes are not harmful but many women are self-conscious about them. About half of the women who reported the symptom suffered considerable distress when flushing[9]. Night sweats that regularly and frequently disturb sleep can lead to psychological distress.

It is believed that hot flushes occur because the decline in estrogen precipitates an imbalance of the temperature-controlling mechanisms in the brain[7,10]. This seems to be related more to fluctuations in estrogen levels than to low estrogen levels *per se*. This could explain why vasomotor disturbances are common in the years before and after the menopause, when

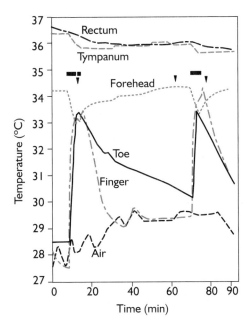

Figure 4.2

Temperature responses to two spontaneous hot flushes (▬▬) and an evoked flush
(■). Reproduced with permission from Molnar GW. Body temperatures during
menopausal hot flashes. *J Appl Physiol* 1975;38:499–503

estrogen levels are erratic, but cease in the later years, when
estrogen levels, although low, have stabilized.

The precise mechanism by which reduced circulating levels of
estrogen cause flushing has yet to be established, and there are
some apparent anomalies. For example, priming with estrogen
seems to be an essential prerequisite for flushing, as young
women with Turner's syndrome (a condition where the ovaries
have not developed or are inactive) have very low circulating
levels of estrogen, but do not have hot flushes. However, if these
women are given estrogen replacement therapy which is later
discontinued, hot flushes can occur and are often a very
distressing problem.

Treatment with HT

Estrogen, administered by the oral, transdermal, nasal or implant routes, relieves hot flushes and sweats provided that sufficiently high blood levels are obtained (Figure 4.3). A recently developed vaginal ring is the only vaginal preparation that is effective systemically. However, it must be used in conjunction with a progestogen, unless the woman has had a hysterectomy. Although some women experience an immediate beneficial response, a gradual improvement over several weeks is more common. For this reason, treatment should be maintained for 3 months before changing the preparation or dose. The elimination

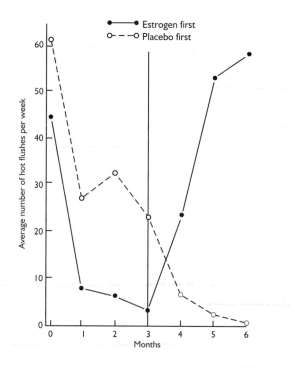

Figure 4.3

Hot flush count during a 6-month cross-over trial with conjugated equine estrogen 1.25 mg daily. Alteration in number of flushes per week after each month of therapy. Reproduced with permission from Coope J, Thompson JM, Poller L. Effects of 'natural estrogen' replacement therapy on menopausal symptoms and blood clotting. *Br Med* J 1975;4:139–43

of hot flushes also improves sleep patterns and this, in turn, can alleviate some of the psychological symptoms resulting from tiredness.

Hot flushes can have a very significant effect on quality of life and cause great embarrassment, especially in the workplace or socially. Although nobody will ever die from a flush, the impact on general well-being and self-esteem should not be underestimated. Flushes are especially distressing in women who are not able to benefit from HT, such as those suffering from breast cancer. These women are usually given the hormone tamoxifen. This is very effective in reducing the risk of cancer spreading to the healthy breast, but a common side-effect is flushing owing to its antiestrogen effect in the brain.

4.4 Alternatives to estrogen for the relief of hot flushes

No other treatment is as effective as estrogen in relieving hot flushes. However, some progestogens (synthetic forms of progesterone) can help. These include norethisterone (5 mg daily[11]) and megestrol acetate (40 mg daily[12]).

In some studies, clonidine has been reported to be helpful in women following breast cancer[13], and recently there have been reports of beneficial effects of drugs that bring about biochemical changes in the brain[14,15].

4.5 Flushes or flashes? Need for uniformity in terminology

It is important to have uniformity in terminology in health studies, and use of the term *flash* instead of *flush* in North America is both regrettable and inappropriate. The *Concise Oxford Dictionary* states that flash implies a sudden transitory blaze, whereas a flush suggests prolonged suffusion with a warm color rather than a transient event.

4.6　Both HT and low-dose vaginal estrogen alleviate urogenital symptoms

Urogenital symptoms

Estrogen deficiency produces gradual atrophy of the tissues of the vagina and urinary tract. These symptoms, unlike hot flushes, do not generally make their appearance until some years after the menopause. Their effects can be very distressing and seriously impair a woman's quality of life.

The earliest symptom to be experienced by the menopausal woman is usually vaginal dryness, which may cause pain or discomfort during intercourse. Estrogen promotes a good blood supply to the vagina and stimulates glands in the cervix and at the entrance to the vagina to produce lubricating secretions. These secretions are fermented by lactobacillus bacteria in the vagina, producing an acid environment, which protects against infection[16]. Thus, in the absence of estrogen, the vagina becomes less acid, which predisposes it to infection. Itching of the vulva and vagina are also common.

Sexual activity has an impact on the health of the vagina. Comparisons of sexually active and abstinent postmenopausal women have shown less vaginal atrophy in those who were active, despite similar blood levels of estrogen in both groups[17].

Many tissues in the urinary tract are sensitive to estrogen. Estrogen maintains the lining of the urethra and, as is the case with the vagina, lack of estrogen leads to an increase in urinary tract infections such as cystitis[18]. Estrogen deficiency may also make the bladder muscle more irritable, and this could explain why menopausal women can suffer from urge incontinence ('overactive bladder'). This is characterized by a very strong desire to empty the bladder, along with an occasional expulsion of urine. However, a direct role of estrogen in this process has not been confirmed. Urge incontinence is exacerbated by urinary infections, which *are* reduced by estrogen. The other common

Table 4.2   Urodynamic findings among climacteric women. Prevalence of urody-namic diagnoses among 285 women attending a menopause clinic. Data from Versi E, Cardozo L, Studd J, et al. Urinary disorders and the menopause. *Menopause* 1995;2:89–95

Urodynamic diagnosis	Prevalence (%)
Normal	59
Genuine stress incontinence	22
Detrusor instability	10
Voiding difficulties	7
Sensory urgency	4

type of incontinence is stress incontinence, in which leakage results from coughing, sneezing, laughing or exercising. Up to one-third of women over the age of 60 suffer from some form of urinary incontinence (Table 4.2). Many factors are involved in the occurrence of this problem, including whether or not a woman has given birth, aging, excessive weight, smoking, certain medications and muscular weakness. Estrogen deficiency is just one factor among many and is not thought to play a significant part in stress incontinence[19].

Treatment with estrogen

These distressing urogenital problems (except those resulting from stress incontinence) can be alleviated with estrogen therapy[19,20] (Table 4.3). The evidence relating to urge incontinence is limited, but a few studies have shown some improvement with estrogen treatment, mainly because of a reduction in urinary tract infections. There are estrogen receptors in the urogenital tract and these react to very low doses of estrogen. However, if the urogenital tract has been without estrogen for some time (as is the case with older women who are just starting HT), these receptors become unresponsive and must be 'kick-started'. Oral estrogen may not do this very well and the

Table 4.3   Summary of estrogen effects in the postmenopausal lower urinary tract. Reproduced from Hoyte L, Versi E. The lower urinary tract in menopause: the contributions of aging and estrogen deficiency. In Studd J, ed. *The Management of the Menopause*. Carnforth, UK: Parthenon Publishing, 2000:151–98

Parameter	Effect of estrogen
Symptoms of urinary incontinence	improved
Genuine stress incontinence (objective diagnosis)	not improved with estrogen alone objective improvement with combination estrogen and α-agonist therapy
Urge incontinence	probably improved
Recurrent urinary tract infections	improved
Urethral pressure profile	inconclusive
Nocturia	improved
Frequency	probably improved
Voiding difficulty	probably improved

receptors need to be stimulated by locally administered vaginal estrogen until a therapeutic response has been achieved after 1 or 2 months. Oral estrogen can then be continued alone.

Once primed, the estrogen receptors in the urogenital tract will respond to low-dose estrogen. Estriol, a natural human estrogen, is particularly suitable for this. It acts specifically on the urogenital tract and does not stimulate the endometrium. Since the bladder and urethra are so close to the vagina, they also benefit from vaginally administered estrogen. Systemic absorption of low doses of estrogen from the vagina is negligible and therefore this route is appropriate for women with contraindications for HT, e.g. breast cancer survivors. However, such low-dose treatment affords no protection against osteoporosis. Once relief of symptoms is obtained, maintenance doses once or twice a week are sufficient, but the problems return if the treatment is stopped. See Appendix for suitable preparations.

Various lubricants are commercially available without prescription, which can be used to counteract vaginal dryness. Vaginal gels create a lubricant film of similar acidity to the normal vagina.

It is unfortunate that many women suffer in silence because they are too embarrassed to ask for help, when the distress caused by these urogenital problems can be so readily alleviated. Unfortunately, if they are not treated early enough, the atrophic changes become less easily corrected by locally administered estrogen.

4.7 The duration of HT depends on the reason for using it

A woman who takes HT to relieve vasomotor symptoms may wish to use it for only a year or two, until the symptoms disappear. Whether the symptoms have stopped permanently can only be determined by stopping the HT and waiting to see if they return. A sudden cessation of HT is more likely to result in withdrawal symptoms than if the dose is gradually reduced over a few weeks. If vaginal dryness remains a problem, the woman may have to stay on HT for as long as she is sexually active. The current thinking is that there are several stages in a woman's life when she can start or restart HT, depending on her needs.

Menopausal symptoms do not last for ever and treatment for 2–4 years is usually sufficient. Many women, however, wish to continue HT in order to enjoy its longer-term benefits. This is when the balance of possible benefits against the risks has to be assessed for each individual.

4.8 HT helps with some aspects of sexual functioning in menopausal women

Women seeking help for menopausal symptoms often raise the issue of sexual problems. Loss of libido and a reduction in the frequency of intercourse and orgasm are common in climacteric women[21] and the question arises as to whether this is due to estrogen deficiency. Human sexuality is highly complex, being affected by psychosocial and emotional, as well as physiological factors. Few population-based studies of the menopause have assessed sexual functioning, and the methodologies of those which have, are open to criticism. One Australian study, which attempted to overcome the limitations of earlier research, measured the relationship between sexuality, mood, menopausal status, hormone levels and psychosocial factors, over a 6-year period in 350 women aged 45–55[22]. The researchers concluded that the effects of female hormones on sexual functioning were relatively insignificant compared with psychosocial factors, particularly the feelings the woman expressed towards her partner. This and other studies suggest that, if loss of sexual interest is caused by urogenital problems such as dry vagina and pain on intercourse, then hormone replacement is helpful. Most studies to date suggest that HT does not have a major direct effect on libido[23]. However, treatment in these studies was with conjugated equine estrogens. Some studies which used estradiol have reported an improvement in sexual interest[24] and it may be that different preparations and delivery routes have different effects.

4.9 Some studies have shown that treatment with a combination of estrogen and testosterone can restore libido in menopausal women

One hormone that has received attention recently for its effects on sex drive is testosterone. Testosterone levels in men are strongly correlated with sex drive, both being at their peak in men in their 20s. Women also produce testosterone and other androgens from the ovaries and adrenal glands, and from the metabolic conversion of other sex steroids. The reduction in ovarian function around the time of the menopause results in decreased testosterone levels. Women who have had their functioning ovaries surgically removed (resulting in a precipitous drop in both estrogen and testosterone) report a reduction in well-being, energy and libido[25]. These are restored more effectively by a combination of estrogen and testosterone than by estrogen alone. Studies in female rhesus monkeys have demonstrated that testosterone exerts its libido-enhancing effect in the brain rather than on peripheral tissues, causing an increase in proceptive behavior, i.e. increased attempts to solicit mounts from the male.

The data relating to women who are androgen-deficient through a natural menopause are much less clear. Implants containing 50 mg of estradiol and 100 mg of testosterone have been used for decades in Britain and Australia for women whose libido remains low despite estrogen therapy. In several studies, women receiving this combined treatment reported significant improvement, not only in libido, but also in energy and well-being[26–28]. However, several placebo-controlled studies measuring sexual interest or intercourse frequency as outcomes have demonstrated no effect. More research needs to be done to clarify a difficult area of study.

Testosterone is not suitable for oral administration because of a direct effect on liver function that could be detrimental to health. For this reason, testosterone is usually given by intramuscular injection or implant. Transdermal patches and gels are currently being evaluated as an alternative route of administration and as possible therapy for reduced libido in both men and women.

As might be expected, research into the beneficial effects of testosterone on libido has aroused considerable interest among women. However, some authorities urge caution[29]. As already stated, human sexuality involves an intricate web of physiological, psychosocial and emotional factors, and for many women, libido is unlikely to be effectively managed by hormones alone.

Other effects of testosterone in women

1) Estrogen/testosterone combinations have recently been shown to increase the bone mineral density of post-menopausal women more than estrogen alone. While estrogen prevents bone loss, this combination increases it by 2–4%.

2) Estrogen replacement therapy has a potential cardioprotective effect by reducing cholesterol levels and improving arterial blood flow (see Sections 6.4 and 6.5). Given by the oral route, combined estrogen/testosterone is less effective in reducing cholesterol than estrogen alone, due to metabolism in the liver, but non-oral routes do not appear to have this disadvantage.

3) Testosterone does not alter the endometrial-stimulating effects of estrogen, indicating that a progestogen is still required.

4) About 20% of women treated with testosterone grow more hair on the chin and upper lip. This increases with the dose of testosterone and is reversible on stopping therapy.

5) Acne, greasy skin and voice changes are rarely a problem.

4.10   HT improves skin quality

Skin is composed of two layers, the outer layer or epidermis, which is constantly being renewed by cells from the underlying dermis. The dermis contains sweat glands, hair follicles and blood vessels, and a large quantity of fibrous tissue, mostly comprised of collagen. Collagen is a major constituent of skin and bone, and is responsible for the skin's resilience and thickness. It is produced by cells called fibroblasts, which have estrogen receptors. Estrogen stimulates the production of collagen by the fibroblasts, and also promotes chemical changes that increase the amount of water in the dermis, giving the skin a firm appearance.

The decline of estrogen at the menopause results in a decrease in collagen, skin thickness and water retention, and many women find that their skin becomes dry and flaky. Some 30% of skin collagen is lost in the first 5 years after the menopause, and this loss mirrors what is happening to bone collagen at this time (see Sections 5.3–5.5). The correlation between susceptibility to osteoporotic fractures and thin, transparent skin was noticed as long as 60 years ago[30].

Several studies have shown that estrogen replacement restores skin collagen and thickness to premenopausal levels, improves skin hydration and limits the loss of skin elasticity, which occurs with age[31-33] (Figure 4.4). However, evidence that it prevents wrinkles is limited.

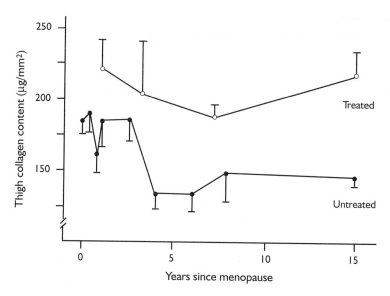

Figure 4.4

Collagen content at the thigh region in untreated ($n = 148$) and estrogen-treated ($n = 59$) postmenopausal women. Reproduced from reference 33 with permission

Nevertheless, there are obvious cosmetic implications for these effects of estrogen, which should be seen as a bonus of HT rather than as the reason to take it. The apparent prolonged sexuality and youthfulness of those mature women in public life who ascribe their age-defying appearance to HT should not be allowed to influence women's choices.

References

1. Lieblum SR, Swartzman LC. Women's attitudes toward the menopause: an update. *Maturitas* 1985;8:47–56

2. Matthews KA, Wing RR, Kuller LH, *et al*. Influences of natural menopause on psychological characteristics and symptoms of mid-aged healthy women. *J Consult Clin Psychol* 1990;58:345–51

3. Van Keep P, Kellerans J. The impact of socio-cultural factors on symptom formation. *Psychother Psychosom* 1974;23:251–63

4. McKinley SM, Jefferys M. The menopausal syndrome. *Br J Prev Soc Med* 1974;28:108–15

5. Campbell S, Whitehead M. Estrogen therapy and the menopausal syndrome. *Clin Obstet Gynecol* 1977;1:31–47

6. Coope J, Thompson JM, Poller L. Effects of 'natural estrogen' replacement therapy on menopausal symptoms and blood clotting. *Br Med J* 1975;4:139–43

7. Sturdee DW, Gokhale LS. The hot flush. In Brincat M, ed. *HT and the Skin*. Carnforth, UK: Parthenon Publishing, 2001: 85–109

8. MacLennan A, Lester S, Moore V. Oral estrogen replacement therapy versus placebo for hot flushes: a systematic review. *Climacteric* 2001;4:58–74

9. Porter M, Penney GC, Russell D, Templeton A. A population based survey of women's experience of the menopause. *Br J Obstet Gynaecol* 1996;103:1025–8

10. Meldrum DL, De Fazio J, Erlik Y, *et al.* Pituitary hormones during the menopausal hot flush. *Obstet Gynecol* 1984;64:752–6

11. Paterson ME. A randomised double-blind cross-over trial into the effect of norethisterone on climacteric symptoms and biochemical profiles. *Br J Obstet Gynaecol* 1982;89:464–72

12. Farish E, Barnes JF, O'Donoghue F, *et al.* The role of megestrol acetate as an alternative to conventional hormone replacement therapy. *Climacteric* 2000;3:125–34

13. Pandya KJ, Raubertas RF, Flynn PJ, *et al.* Oral clonidine in post-menopausal patients with breast cancer experiencing tamoxifen-induced hot flashes: a University of Rochester Cancer Center Community Clinical Oncology Program study. *Ann Intern Med* 2000;132:788–93

14. Stearns V, Isaacs C, Rowland J, *et al.* A pilot trial assessing the efficacy of paroxetine hydrochloride (Paxil) in controlling hot flushes in breast cancer survivors. *Ann Oncol* 2000;11:17–22

15. Loprinzi CL, Kugler JW, Sloan JA, *et al.* Venlafaxine in the management of hot flushes in survivors of breast cancer: a randomised controlled trial. *Lancet* 2000;356:2059–63

16. Milsom I, Arvidsson L, Ekeland P, Molander U, Eriksson O. Factors affecting vaginal cytology, pH and bacterial flora in elderly women. *Acta Obstet Gynecol Scand* 1993;72:286–91

17. Bachmann GA, Leiblum SR, Kemmann E, Colburn DW, Swartzman L, Shelden R. Sexual expression and its determinants in the post-menopausal woman. *Maturitas* 1984;6:19–29

18. Molander U, Milsom I, Ekelund P, Mellström D. An epidemiological study of urinary incontinence and related urogenital symptoms in elderly women. *Maturitas* 1990;12:51–60

19. Cardozo LD, Kelleher CJ. Sex hormones, the menopause and urinary problems. *Gynecol Endocrinol* 1995;9:75–84

20. Molander U, Milsom I, Ekelund P, Mellström D, Eriksson O. Effect of oral estriol on vaginal flora and cytology and urogenital symptoms in the postmenopause. *Maturitas* 1990;12:113–20

21. Hallström T. Sexuality of women in middle age: the Gotteburg study. *J Biosoc Soc* 1979;6(Suppl):165–75

22. Dennerstein L, Lehert P, Burger H, Dudley E. Factors affecting sexual functioning of women in the mid-life years. *Climacteric* 1999;2:254–62

23. Myers LS, Dixon J, Morrissette M, Carmichael M, Davidson JM. Effects of estrogen, androgen and progesterone on sexual psychophysiology and behaviour in postmenopausal women. *J Clin Endocrinol Metab* 1990;70:1124–31

24. McCoy NL. Sexual issues for postmenopausal women. *Top Geriatr Rehab* 1997;12:28–39

25. Kaplan HS, Owett T. The female androgen deficiency syndrome. *Sex Marital Ther* 1993;19:3–24

26. Brincat M, Magos A, Studd JWW, *et al*. Subcutaneous hormone implants for the control of climacteric symptoms: a prospective study. *Lancet* 1984;1:16–18

27. Burger HG, Hailles J, Menelaus M, *et al*. The management of persistent menopausal symptoms with estradiol testosterone implants: clinical, lipid and hormonal results. *Maturitas* 1984;6:351–8

28. Burger HG, Hailles J, Nelson J, *et al*. Effects of combined implants of estradiol and testosterone on libido in postmenopausal women. *Lancet* 1987;294:936–7

29. Levine SB. Women's sexual capacities at mid-life. In Eskin BA, ed. *The Menopause: Comprehensive Management*, 4th edn. Carnforth, UK: Parthenon Publishing, 2000:53–61

30. Albright F, Smith PH, Richardson AM. Postmenopausal osteoporosis: its clinical features. *J Am Med Assoc* 1941;116:465–74

31. Brincat M, Moniz CF, Studd JWW, *et al*. Long-term effects of the menopause and sex hormones on skin thickness. *Br J Obstet Gynaecol* 1985;92:256–9

32. Pierard GE, Letawe C, Dowlati A, *et al*. Effect of hormone replacement therapy for menopause on mechanical properties of skin. *J Am Geriatr Soc* 1995;43:662–5

33. Brincat M, ed. *HT and the Skin*. Carnforth, UK: Parthenon Publishing, 2001

Chapter 5

HT and osteoporosis

5.1   The rates of osteoporosis and fracture rise rapidly after the menopause

Bone mass starts to decline at a surprisingly young age, at about 30 years in both sexes, and continues throughout the rest of life. As life expectancy increases bones have longer to degenerate and the likelihood of osteoporotic fracture rises with age. Women are much more at risk of fracture than men for three reasons:

(1)   Their peak bone mass is less than that in men;

(2)   They live, on average, longer than men and so have a longer period of bone loss;

(3)   Most significantly, their rate of bone loss exceeds that in men once the menopause is reached and estrogen levels diminish.

The lifetime risk of fracture for men and women at the age of 50 years is shown in Table 5.1, and a schematic representation of life-time changes in bone mass in men and women is provided in Figure 5.1.

Table 5.1   Lifetime risk of fracture (%) at age 50 years[2]

	Men	Women
Spine	2	11
Wrist	2	13
Hip	3	14

Estrogen plays an important role in building bone mass during adolescence and in maintaining it in adulthood. To some extent, men are protected by their continuing secretion of testosterone and thus they do not experience the same rapid deterioration as women until they reach their 70s.

5.2   Bone is constantly broken down and reformed

Bone consists of a strong but flexible collagen matrix permeated with minerals (mainly calcium phosphate), and well supplied

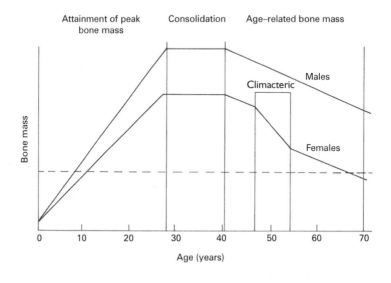

Figure 5.1

Schematic representation of lifetime changes in bone mass. From reference 1 with permission

with blood vessels. It is not inert, but is constantly being remodelled, i.e. broken down and renewed, in response to varying demands put upon the skeleton. This process ensures that bones heal after fracture, increase in mass as a result of regular exercise, and that surplus bone is removed during a spell of immobilization.

Remodelling results from the activity of two types of cell. *Osteoclasts* break down old bone, dissolving its minerals and proteins, some of which are then excreted by the kidneys. This process is known as bone *resorption*. The other cell type (*osteoblasts*) is responsible for rebuilding bone from raw materials such as amino acids and calcium, which must be provided in the diet. For a schematic representation of the bone remodelling process, see Figure 5.2.

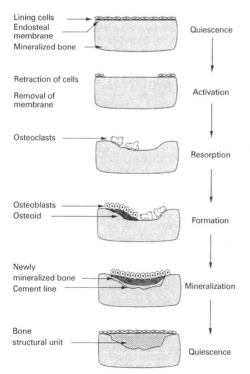

Figure 5.2

Schematic representation of bone remodelling. Reproduced from Compston JE. Bone morphology: quality, quantity and strength. In Shaw RW, ed. *Advances in Reproductive Endocrinology*, Vol. 8, *Oestrogen Deficiency: Causes and Consequences*. Carnforth, UK: Parthenon Publishing Group, 1996:63–84

The entire skeleton undergoes complete remodelling over a period of 7–10 years in mature adults, and over 2–3 years in children and young adults. The shafts of the long bones consist of tightly packed columns of *compact* bone, while the bone ends have a more open, honeycomb structure called *trabecular* bone. Trabecular bone is also found in the spine, and in parts of the skeleton which do not bear much weight, e.g. the pelvis and shoulder blade. Remodelling is more rapid in trabecular bone than in the dense bone of the shafts, making the former more susceptible to osteoporotic degradation. Not only does osteoporosis involve a loss of mass but the architecture of the bone changes, with numerous structural cross-links being lost, drastically reducing its strength (Figure 5.3).

The commonest sites of fracture are the trabecular bone at the top of the femur (hip fracture), the vertebrae of the spine (vertebral crush fracture; Figure 5.4) and the radius near the wrist.

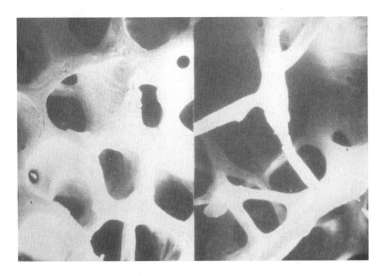

Figure 5.3

Healthy and osteoporotic trabecular bone. Reproduced, with permission, from Dempster D, Shane E, Horbert R, *et al.* A simple method for correlative scanning electron microscopy of human iliac crest biopsies. *Am J Bone Min Res* 1986;1:15–21

5.3 Over 40% of women will suffer at least one fracture caused by osteoporosis

Women lose 50% of their skeleton by age 70, while men lose only 25% by age 90. Without estrogen, female bone density typically decreases by about 2% per year in the spine and 1% per year in the hip, although in some unlucky women the loss is as much as 10% and 5%, respectively. These 'fast losers' are indistinguishable from their more fortunate sisters, because osteoporosis shows no symptoms until a fracture occurs. A 10% loss of bone approximately doubles the risk of fracture. In severe cases, repeated vertebral compression fractures may result in thoracic kyphosis, commonly known as 'Dowager's hump' (Figure 5.5).

The incidence of the disease is high (Figure 5.6) and is predicted to increase. Osteoporosis constitutes one of the most serious

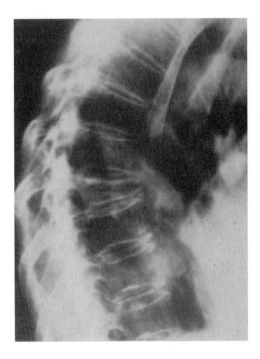

Figure 5.4

X-ray showing vertebral osteoporosis and wedge compression fracture

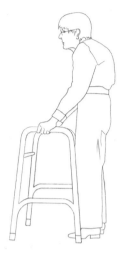

Figure 5.5

Thoracic kyphosis (Dowager's hump)

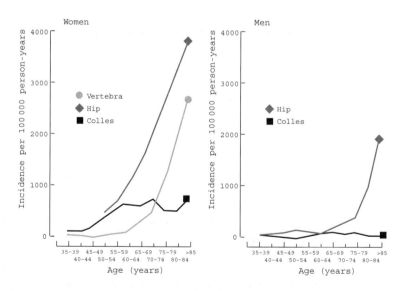

Figure 5.6

Incidence of osteoporotic fracture in men and women. Reproduced with permission from Riggs BL, Melton LJ. Involutional osteoporosis. *N Engl J Med* 1986;314:1676–86. Copyright © 1986 Massachusetts Medical Society. All rights reserved

health problems currently faced by industrialized countries (Table 5.2).

5.4 Estrogen is one of several regulatory factors involved in bone remodelling

The remodelling process is controlled by a complex and, as yet, poorly understood mechanism, which includes:

Table 5.2   Some statistics concerning osteoporotic fractures

- In the UK, approximately 200 000 people per year suffer fractures of the vertebrae, hip and forearm

- Approximately seven million women are postmenopausal and over three million will eventually suffer at least one osteoporotic fracture in their lifetime

- The annual cost to the Health Service is around £500 million

- In the United States at least 1.3 million fractures per year are attributable to osteoporosis

- It is estimated that 4–6 million women in the United States have osteoporosis, and a further 13–17 million have low bone density at the hip

- The cost of health care for osteoporotic fractures was estimated in 1995 to be $US13.8 billion

- In some countries, 20% of hospital beds are occupied by people with hip fractures

- One-quarter of hip fracture patients need long-term nursing care and one-third never regain full independence

- 40% of hip fracture patients still cannot walk independently after 1 year and 60% have problems with some aspect of independent living. This has knock-on effects for carers and support services

- Fractures of the vertebrae cause significant complications such as back pain, height loss and curvature of the spine

(1) *Calcitonin*, a hormone secreted by the thyroid gland which inhibits bone resorption;

(2) *Vitamin D*, which promotes calcium absorption and mineralization of bone;

(3) *Parathyroid hormone*, which stimulates bone resorption;

(4) *Estrogen*, which stimulates bone formation, possibly by increasing calcitonin secretion[3] and inhibiting the resorptive effect of parathyroid hormone[4]. Estrogen may operate via a large number of growth factors, this being an area that requires further research.

Parathyroid hormone, therefore, promotes osteoporosis, whereas calcitonin, vitamin D and estrogen are protective. In normally menstruating women, this complicated system is, more or less, in equilibrium. The menopausal fall in estrogen levels removes an important check on the activities of parathyroid hormone, and the rate of resorption increases. However, the rate at which new bone is created remains the same, with the net result of bone loss.

5.5 HT is an effective preventative treatment for osteoporosis

The protective effect of estrogen on the skeleton was first observed in the 1940s, when it was found to reduce height loss in postmenopausal women[5]. The development of better methods of measuring bone density revealed that bone depletion in post-menopausal women was widespread, and by the 1970s the preventative role of estrogen had become evident. Since then, numerous studies have confirmed that estrogen, in the doses used in HT (Table 5.3), maintains bone in 90% of estrogen-deficient women. The addition of a progestogen does not diminish the effect of estrogen, and several studies have shown a potentiating effect[6,7]. One of the most significant long-term studies carried

Table 5.3   Daily doses of estrogen needed to protect the skeleton

Oral estradiol	1–2 mg
Conjugated equine estrogens	0.3–0.625 mg
Transdermal estradiol	25–50 µg

out to date is the Postmenopausal Estrogen/Progestin Interventions (PEPI) trial[8]. This trial assigned women to different estrogen/progestogen treatments and measured, among other parameters of postmenopausal health, the alteration in bone density after 36 months. The women allocated to the placebo (dummy) treatment lost almost 2% of their bone density in the hip and spine, whereas treated women gained 3.5–5% in the spine and nearly 2% at the hip. The greatest increases were seen in those who took continuous progestogen with the estrogen.

Many other studies support these results and estrogen is widely considered to be the most effective and natural means of preventing bone loss and reducing the prevalence of osteoporotic fractures in women. Although both the oral and transdermal routes are effective in preserving bone[9,10] (Figure 5.7), studies have shown that after an initial increase for 2–3 years, bone density reaches a plateau, after which there is a slight decline. However, this decline is much less than is seen in women not taking HT. Subcutaneous implants, which produce a higher level of estrogen in the blood, may have a greater effect as the response appears to be related to the level of estrogen[11] in the circulation. Thus, women who have been having estradiol implants for many years generally have much greater bone density than those who have been using other routes.

The bone-protective effects of estrogen have been observed in menopausal women, in women with established osteoporosis, and even in elderly women for whom low doses of estrogen are

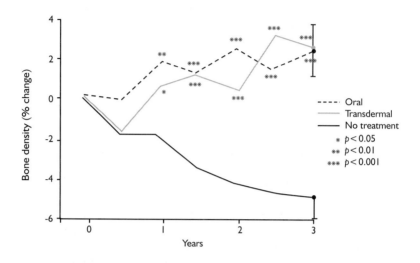

Figure 5.7

Effects on femoral neck bone density of oral and transdermal estrogen therapy compared with no estrogen treatment. Reproduced with permission from Hillard TC, Whitcroft SJ, Marsh MS, *et al.* Long-term effects of transdermal and oral hormone replacement therapy on postmenopausal bone loss. *Osteoporos Int* 1994;4:341–8.

effective (Table 5.2). Thus, it is never too late to start HT. Even short periods of estrogen therapy have been effective in preventing hip fractures in women over 75 years of age[12]. Younger women who have risk factors for osteoporosis (Table 5.4) should start treatment at the menopause, before significant bone loss occurs. However, once women stop their course of treatment, bone loss begins again. Estrogen is protective only for as long as it is used. Therefore, for estrogen to be effective in preventing osteoporosis, the treatment should be long-term, that is, of at least 10 years' duration.

Table 5.4   Contributory factors for osteoporosis

- *Genetic factors.* Women whose mothers had a hip fracture are more likely to exhibit low bone density. Black women have a genetically endowed higher bone density than white

- *Prolonged failure of menstruation* (amenorrhea) for any reason other than pregnancy indicates a shortage of estrogen. This may happen as a result of anorexia, excessive sports or dance training, hard drug use or an underlying hormonal disorder

- *Hysterectomy with conserved ovaries.* In this situation, the ovaries may stop functioning a few years earlier than expected, and this may go undetected. The reason for this is not known, but it increases the risk of osteoporosis

- *Long-term use of corticosteroids* has an inhibitory effect on bone development and calcium absorption in the gut. There is evidence that the use of inhalers by asthmatics, which exposes them to small systemic doses of corticosteroids over a long period, produces some decrease in bone mineral density[13]. The effects of corticosteroids on bone mineral density can be reduced by prophylactic therapy with calcium and vitamin D[14]

- *Calcium or vitamin D* deficiency may result from an inadequate diet or exposure to sunlight, or a medical condition which inhibits absorption of nutrients, e.g. Crohn's disease

- *Lack of physical exercise.* The bone density of athletes is higher than that of the general population[15]. Prolonged bed rest causes bone loss[16]. Weight-bearing exercise has a modest effect on bone density[17]. This is illustrated by amenorrheic (and therefore estrogen-deficient) ballet dancers or athletes who suffer bone loss despite vigorous exercise regimens. Exercise also improves muscle strength and co-ordination, and reduces the likelihood of falls

- *Smoking.* The risk of hip fracture is higher in smokers, and increases with cigarette consumption. Smoking negates the protective effects of estrogen on the skeleton[18,19] by activating an enzyme which converts estrogen to a metabolite with antiestrogen effects. Thus, smoking not only lowers estrogen levels but also blocks the effect of the remaining estrogen. Giving up smoking decreases the risk but the effects are not seen until 10 years after stopping. Smokers tend to have an earlier menopause and are estrogen-deficient for longer

- *Alcohol.* Chronic alcohol abuse is associated with reduced bone mass and an increased risk of fractures. Moderate consumption (one or two units per day) does not appear to affect bone mass[20]

5.6   Treatments other than HT are available for osteoporosis

HT is widely considered to be the most logical and the best treatment for conserving bone mass, but some women are reluctant or unable to use it. Fortunately, some alternatives are available.

Bisphosphonates

The bisphosphonates are a family of synthetic compounds which inhibit bone resorption. They do this by forming a coating over the inner surfaces of trabecular bone, protecting it from attack by the osteoclasts (cells that break down bone). Several studies have also shown that bisphosphonates increase bone mineral density in the spine and hip[21,22]. However, because their mode of action inhibits the entire remodelling process, bone treated with bisphosphonates loses its ability to respond to environmental stimuli, which may weaken it in the long term. Bisphosphonates are long-acting and can have a cumulative effect, causing bone demineralization. This can be minimized by intermittent use. A further disadvantage is that gastrointestinal side-effects are common. Recent introduction of a once per week preparation of alendronate should improve patient acceptability.

The combination of HT with alendronate has an additive effect and provides greater improvement in bone mineral density than either therapy alone. Combination therapy may be the best option for those with severe osteoporosis or who have not responded satisfactorily to single therapy[23].

Calcitonin

Calcitonin is a natural hormone produced by the thyroid gland, which inhibits the activity of the bone-dissolving cells and thus reduces bone resorption. Interestingly, low calcitonin levels have not been found in people with osteoporosis. Nevertheless, administration of calcitonin has been shown to reduce the incidence of fractures in the hip and spine by up to two-thirds[24]. It is also a potent pain-killer. Calcitonin is an expensive product to manufacture, and can only be taken by injection or used as a nasal spray. For these reasons, it is not considered to be a viable alternative to estrogen.

Raloxifene

Raloxifene is a selective estrogen receptor modulator or SERM (see Section 2.7). It mimics the action of estrogen in some tissues, including bone. It has been shown to inhibit resorption, increase bone density in the hip and spine, and reduce vertebral fractures by 30–50%[25]. However, the same study showed no reduction in hip fracture with raloxifene treatment and the authors speculate that the drug may have to be used for 5 years before significant fracture reduction is seen at this site. Raloxifene is licensed in the United States and the UK for the treatment of osteoporosis.

Tibolone

Tibolone is a synthetic steroid with estrogenic, progestogenic and androgenic properties. It is as effective as HT in alleviating climacteric symptoms and has been shown to increase bone mass in the spine and hip, although no data are available regarding its effect on fracture risk[26].

Calcium and vitamin D

Adequate calcium intake is necessary throughout life to promote peak bone mass and maintain bone health. There has been some debate about the value of calcium supplements in reducing osteoporosis after the menopause, but studies in elderly people have confirmed that a high intake (1500 mg per day) is protective[27]. This high dose seems to operate by raising blood calcium to a level which inhibits the production of parathyroid hormone. As a result, resorption of bone is reduced. Lower intakes of calcium do not inhibit parathyroid hormone and, therefore, are not effective. Realistically, this amount of calcium is unlikely to be supplied from dietary sources and supplementation is advisable.

Vitamin D is needed to absorb calcium from food and to promote bone mineralization. It is obtained from milk fats and fish oils, or from exposure of the skin to sunlight. With the current popularity of low-fat diets and the need to avoid excessive sun exposure, it may be expedient to take vitamin D supplements to ensure an adequate intake.

Calcium and vitamin D cannot replace HT and other therapies as a treatment for osteoporosis, but they provide a first line of defence.

Natural progesterone

A natural progesterone cream has been widely promoted in the media as a natural alternative to HT for preventing osteoporosis or as a supplement to estrogen[28]. However, there are no controlled data to support any clinical benefit and recent reports have shown that absorption into the circulation is minimal[29,30].

5.7 Strategies to reduce the risk of fracture

Hip and wrist fractures usually result from a fall. The following measures can help to reduce the risk of falling:

(1) HT helps to maintain the sense of balance and thus reduces the incidence of stumbling and falls;

(2) Avoiding stairs and reducing opportunities for tripping and losing balance in the home;

(3) Minimizing sedative medications and avoiding drugs which impair balance;

(4)   Regular exercise to maintain muscle strength and reduce the tendency to fall;

(5)   Staying indoors during icy conditions;

(6)   External hip protectors for the vulnerable[31].

5.8   The risk of osteoporosis can be reduced if optimum bone mass is attained in youth

Since bone quality declines for many more years than it improves, it is important to optimize its growth while it is possible to do so (Figure 5.1). The significance of adolescence and young adulthood as a time to build bone cannot be overemphasized. Over 50% of the skeletal mass is laid down during puberty, and after the age of 30 there is no opportunity to make up any deficit.

Unfortunately, modern lifestyles are not conducive for optimal bone growth during this period. The decline in manual work, the ubiquity of the motor car, and the downgrading of sport in the school curriculum mean that only a minority of adolescents exercise sufficiently to develop their bones to their full potential. In addition, media and peer pressures with regard to body weight cause many young women to restrict their food intake to below that needed to provide an adequate supply of bone-building nutrients (children need up to 1000 mg and adolescent girls up to 1600 mg calcium daily). Smoking, which reduces the beneficial effects of estrogen and hastens the menopause by about 2 years, is also on the increase among young women. It is a sad fact that osteoporosis is rising at a faster rate than can be explained by longevity alone, and is affecting increasingly younger women.

While adverse conditions have a greater effect on younger women, other contributory factors for osteoporosis apply at any age. These may be related to genetic inheritance, to an underlying medical condition or to lifestyle (Table 5.4).

5.9   Bone density measurement is an effective means of monitoring osteoporosis

Osteoporosis is an insidious process, showing no symptoms until a fracture occurs. The usual method of diagnosing osteoporosis and following its progress is by measuring bone density. This is done using a non-invasive technique called densitometry. There are a number of different scanning systems of varying sophistication in use, the best available method being known as a dual-energy X-ray absorptiometry (DEXA) scan, which can provide an accurate measurement of bone density in the hip and spine (Figure 5.8). This can be repeated every 2 years to monitor either the effectiveness of treatment or the progress of the disease. The result obtained by this technique allows a

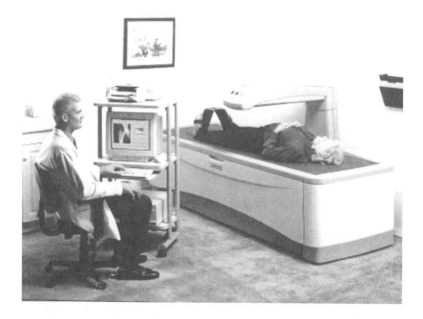

Figure 5.8

A dual-energy X-ray absorptiometry (DEXA) scanner. Reproduced with permission from the National Osteoporosis Society (www.nos.org.uk)

comparison to be made with the average density of the young adult population (T-score). This score is directly related to fracture risk, with values between −1 and −2.5 indicating osteopenia (bone density is reduced but not yet osteoporotic), and values of less than −2.5 being indicative of osteoporosis with its attendant four-fold increase in fracture risk.

Another means of monitoring bone is to carry out blood tests for various biochemical markers, which measure the rate of bone resorption. Although these tests cannot diagnose low bone mineral density, they may provide some indication of whether treatment is working. More reliable biochemical markers are needed.

5.10 There is some debate within the medical profession about who should be referred for densitometry, and how often

Routine screening of all menopausal women would be expensive. Without it, however, many women with lowered bone density would be not be diagnosed and treated. Women with risk factors should be screened, but the question remains: does being menopausal constitute a sufficient risk factor in itself? Women themselves may force the hand of the medical profession. As awareness of the risks of osteoporosis grows, fuelled by the work of organizations such as the National Osteoporosis Society (www.nos.org.uk), more symptomless and otherwise risk-free menopausal women are initiating discussions with their doctors as to the best way forward.

It has been suggested that women willing to take HT need not be screened. However, a number of studies have indicated that some women do not maintain their bone mineral density on 'standard' doses of HT. It would be tempting to attribute this to non-compliance but, taking this into account, one study has shown that 12% of the treated group continued to lose bone[32]. Unless some form of screening is done, such women will be under the mistak-

Table 5.5   Guidelines for the referral of women for bone density screening[33]

- Any estrogen-deficient woman who would want treatment if found to be osteoporotic or osteopenic

- Patients with X-rays suggesting osteoporosis, or with height loss and/or low-impact fracture

- Patients who have a treatable medical condition predisposing to osteoporosis (other than estrogen deficiency)

- Patients about to start oral corticosteroids for 6 months or longer, and those already receiving doses greater than 7.5 mg of prednisolone or equivalent

- Estrogen-deficient women under the age of 45 years with amenorrhea

- Patients with a family history of osteoporosis in a first-degree relative

en impression that their HT is protecting them from osteoporosis. Ideally, this could be determined by a simple blood test, but these are not yet reliable enough.

This raises the question of how often women should be screened. Should they be followed up at regular intervals to monitor the progress of the disease or the effectiveness of treatment, as is routinely done with other potentially serious conditions, such as raised blood pressure? The development of cheaper and more mobile equipment such as ultrasound will make monitoring more readily available and cost-effective.

Suggestions from the British Menopause Society[33] regarding screening are shown in Table 5.5. Similar indications from the American National Osteoporosis Foundation can be found on the Internet (www.nof.org). Despite the debate, the current situation is that relatively few women are being referred, even those with known risk factors, and densitometers are not utilized to their full capacity.

5.11 Estrogen replacement therapy needs to be continued for at least 10 years to combat osteoporosis

The protective effects of estrogen last only as long as the estrogen is taken. Once it is stopped, bone loss accelerates just as it did at the climacteric. Some authorities recommend that estrogen should be taken for at least 10 years, starting at the menopause. This gives rise to three considerations:

(1) There is an increased risk of breast cancer with long-term HT use (see Section 8.6). Most women would probably accept the tiny increases in risk arising after 5 years' use; however, many are likely to be anxious about the risk after 10 years' exposure (six extra cases per 1000 women).

(2) If sequential therapy is used, women are faced with the disagreeable prospect of continuing to have periods until they reach the age of 60. This can be avoided by use of the newer continuous combined regimens or tibolone, and it is the responsibility of doctors to offer these to their patients if appropriate.

(3) It is often assumed that this 10-year treatment period will 'buy' enough bone protection to protect the skeleton into old age. However, after 10 years, when the treatment is discontinued, the woman will be about 60 years of age. Bone loss will advance inexorably and, by the time she is 75 years of age (after which most hip fractures occur), there will be little difference between her bones and those of a woman who has never taken HT[34]. A solution might be to take HT for about 5 years to cover acute menopausal symptoms, and then start the 10-year programme between the ages of 60 and 65, by which time the breast cancer risk will have returned to baseline. It has been predicted that there is only a 2–6% difference in bone density at the age

of 85 between women who have used estrogen continuously since the menopause, and those who started at the age of 65[35]. This concept of two periods in a woman's life when she is a candidate for HT, at the perimenopause and again in her 60s, is worth considering. Another option is to use raloxifene or one of the other available bone-preserving treatments such as bisphosphonates. Ideally, these clinical decisions should be made in the light of each individual's bone density and exposure to risk factors.

5.12   What is the evidence that HT prevents fractures?

There is no doubt that osteoporosis is a major cause of fracture, but there is little scientific evidence that HT reduces the incidence of fractures[36,37]. HT does reduce bone loss but there has only been one properly controlled study (WHI) that has been continued for long enough to demonstrate a significant reduction in fractures, especially of the hip[38]. Such studies are very expensive and difficult to organize, but further useful data may become available from other ongoing trials that are primarily investigating the effects of HT on heart disease.

References

1.   Compston JE. Osteoporosis. *Clin Endocrinol* 1990;33:653–82

2.   Cooper C. Femoral neck bone density and fracture risk. *Osteoporosis Int* 1996;6(Suppl 3):24–6

3.   Stevenson JC, Abeyasekera G, Hillyard CJ, *et al.* Calcitonin and the calcium regulating hormones in postmenopausal women: effect of estrogens. *Lancet* 1981;1:693–5

4. De Cherney A. Physiologic and pharmacologic effects of estrogen and progestins on bone. *J Reprod Med* 1993;38(Suppl 12):1007–14

5. Albright F, Smith PH, Richardson AM. Postmenopausal osteoporosis: its clinical features. *J Am Med Assoc* 1941;116:2465–74

6. Abdalla HI, Hart DM, Lindsay R, Leggate I, Hooke A. Prevention of bone loss in postmenopausal women by norethisterone. *Obstet Gynecol* 1985;66:789–92

7. Christiansen C, Riis BJ. 17βeta-estradiol and continuous norethisterone: a unique treatment for established osteoporosis in elderly women. *N Engl J Med* 1990;71:836–41

8. The Writing Group for the PEPI Trial. Effects of estrogen/progestin regimens on heart disease risk factors in postmenopausal women. *J Am Med Assoc* 1995;273:199–208

9. Stevenson JC, Cust MP, Gangar KF, *et al*. Effects of transdermal vs oral hormone replacement therapy on bone density in spine and proximal femur in postmenopausal women. *Lancet* 1990;336:265–9

10. Lindsay R, Hart DM, Clark DM. The minimum effective dose of estrogen for prevention of postmenopausal bone loss. *Obstet Gynecol* 1984;63:759–63

11. Studd JWW, Holland EFN, Lever AT, Smith RMJ. The dose response of percutaneous estradiol implants on the skeletons of postmenopausal women. *J Obstet Gynecol* 1994;101:787–91

12. Cauley JA, Seeley DG, Ensrud K, *et al.*, for the Study of Osteoporotic Fractures Research Group. Estrogen replacement

therapy and fractures in older women. *Ann Intern Med* 1995;122:9–16

13. Wong CA, Walsh LJ, Smith CJ, *et al*. Inhaled corticosteroid use and bone-mineral density in patients with asthma. *Lancet* 2000;355:1399–403

14. Singh RF, Muskelly CC. Inhaled corticosteroid-induced bone loss and preventive strategies. *J Am Osteopath Assoc* 2000;100(Suppl 7):S14–17

15. Dook JE, James C, Henderson NK, Price RI. Exercise and bone mineral density in mature female athletes. *Med Sci Sports Exerc* 1997;29:291–6

16. Donaldson CL, Hulley SB, Vogel JM, *et al*. Effect of prolonged bed rest on bone mineral. *Metab Clin Exp* 1970;19:1071–84

17. Kohrt WM, Sneed DB, Slatopolsky E, Birge SJ. Additive effects of weight-bearing exercise and estrogen on bone mineral density in older women. *J Bone Miner Res* 1995;10:1303–11

18. Krall EA, Dawson-Highes B. Smoking and bone loss among postmenopausal women. *J Bone Min Res* 1991;6:331–8

19. Seeman E, Allen T. Risk factors for osteoporosis. *Aust NZ J Med* 1989;19:69–75

20. Holbrook TL, Barrett-Connor E. A prospective study of alcohol consumption and bone mineral density. *Br Med J* 1993;306:1506–9

21. Watts NB, Becker P. Alendronate increases spine and hip bone mineral density in women with postmenopausal osteoporosis

who failed to respond to intermittent cyclical etidronate. *Bone* 1999;24:65–8

22. Devogelaer JP, Broll H, Correa-Rotter R, *et al*. Oral alendronate induces progressive increases in bone mass of the hip, spine and total body over 3 years in women with osteoporosis *Bone* 1996;18:141–50

23. Greenspan SL, Resnick NM, Parker RA. Combination therapy with hormone replacement and alendronate for prevention of bone loss in elderly women: a randomized controlled trial. *J Am Med Assoc* 2003;289:2525–33

24. Overgaard K, Hansen MA, Jensen SB, Christiansen C. Effect of calcitonin given intranasally on bone mass and fracture rates in established osteoporosis: a dose-response study. *Br Med J* 1992;305:556–61

25. Ettinger B, Black DM, Mitlak BH, *et al*. Reduction of vertebral fracture risk in postmenopausal women with osteoporosis treated with raloxifene. Results from a 3-year randomised clinical trial. *J Am Med Assoc* 1999;282:637–45

26. Berning B, Coelingh Bennink HJT, Fauser BCJM. Tibolone and its effects on bone: a review. *Climacteric* 2001;4:120–36

27. Prince R. The calcium controversy revisited: implications of the new data. *Med J Aust* 1993;159:404–7

28. Lee J. Osteoporosis reversed: the role of progesterone. *Int Clin Nutr Rev* 1990;10:384–9

29. Cooper A, Spencer C, Whitehead MI, *et al*. Systemic absorption of micronised progesterone from Progest cream in postmenopausal women. *Lancet* 1998;351:1255–6

30. Wren BG, McFarland L, Edwards P, et al. Effect of sequential transdermal progesterone cream on endometrium, bleeding pattern and plasma and salivary progesterone levels in postmenopausal women. *Climacteric* 2000;3:155–60

31. Lauritzen JB, Petersen MM, Lund B. Effect of external hip protectors on hip fractures. *Lancet* 1993;341:11–13

32. Hillard TC, Whitcroft SJ, Marsh MS, et al. Long-term effects of transdermal and oral hormone replacement therapy on postmenopausal bone loss. *Osteoporosis Int* 1994;4:341–8

33. Rees M, Purdie DW, eds. *Management of the Menopause: The Handbook of the British Menopause Society*. Marlow, UK: BMS Publications, 1997

34. Felson DT, Zhang Y, Hannan MT, Kiel DP, Wilson PW, Anderson JJ. The effect of postmenopausal estrogen therapy on bone density in elderly women. *N Engl J Med* 1993;329:1141–6

35. Ettinger B, Grady D. Maximising the benefit of estrogen therapy for prevention of osteoporosis. *Menopause* 1994;1:19–24

36. Henry D, Robertson J, O'Connell D, Gillespie W. A systematic review of the skeletal effects of estrogen therapy in postmenopausal women. I. An assessment of the quality of randomized trials between 1977 and 1995. *Climacteric* 1998;1:92–111

37. O'Connell D, Robertson J, Henry D, Gillespie W. A systematic review of the skeletal effects of estrogen therapy in postmenopausal women. II. An assessment of treatment effects. *Climacteric* 1998;1:112–13

38. Writing Group for the Women's Health Group Initiative. Risks and benefits of estrogen plus progestin in healthy postmenopausal women. *J Am Med Assoc* 2002;288:321–33

Chapter 6

HT and the cardiovascular system

6.1   Introduction

Theoretically, HT could be a valuable weapon in the fight against heart disease from which about 50% of women die prematurely in Western countries. Estrogen produces favorable changes in many of the biochemical processes associated with an increased risk of heart disease, particularly a reduction in cholesterol levels and a relaxant effect on the arteries. Numerous studies have shown a reduced risk in current or past users of HT, notably the Nurses Health Study from the USA[1], but these have all been observational studies which are vulnerable to bias and especially the 'healthy user effect'. Recent studies of postmenopausal women with established cardiovascular disease (HERS) and women without known cardiovascular disease (WHI), have shown a small increase in mortality in the first year of treatment, and these studies have substantially altered much opinion on the relative merits of HT in protecting from cardiovascular disease.

The addition of a progestogen to HT regimens does not appear to counteract the effects of estrogen on the cardiovascular system. Transdermal estrogen may be a better option for women with some risk factors. The SERM raloxifene has beneficial effects on some cardiovascular disease factors, and a major prospective study on the cardioprotective effects is in progress (RUTH; see section 6.12). Since the HERS and WHI studies, there is a widespread consensus that HT should not be started in women with existing heart disease, but can be continued in those who have been taking it for some time. For women who do not have any apparent risk factors for cardiovascular disease, and who lead a healthy lifestyle, there is no evidence of any cardiovascular benefit from HT.

6.2 The extent of the disease and women's perception of the risk

Cardiovascular disease (CVD), of which coronary heart disease (CHD) is the most frequent, is the most common cause of death in women over the age of 60 years and is uncommon prior to the menopause. In the year 2000, death due to coronary disease occurred in 1022 women below the age of 55, compared with 4600 men (Figure 6.1)[2]. Although the total number of coronary deaths in men and women of all ages is about the same, and as atherosclerosis is a slowly progressive disease, much of this process will have been initiated prior to the menopause[2]. About 50% of all women develop CHD in their lifetime, and 30% will die from the disease, with a further 20% developing a stroke. It is surprising, though, that the public generally perceive that breast cancer is a far more common cause of death in women, whereas the reality is almost exactly opposite to the general perception (Figure 6.2)[3]. Women do, however, tend to develop symptoms of CHD later than men, and functioning ovaries that are producing estrogen seem to provide some degree of protection which is lost at the menopause. The menopause is associated with an increasing incidence of CHD (Figure 6.3)[4].

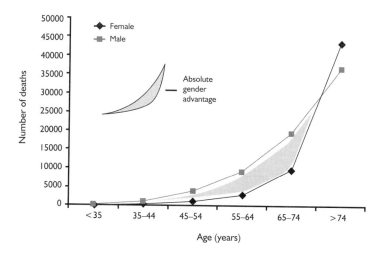

Figure 6.1

Deaths from coronary heart disease in men and women in 2000. Reproduced from reference 2 with permission

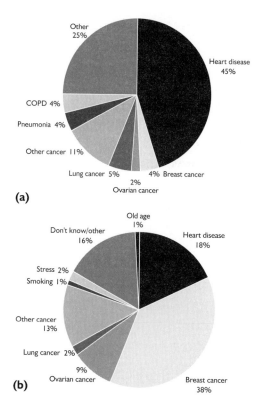

Figure 6.2

Actual leading causes of death in women (a) compared to perceived causes (b). COPD, chronic obstructive pulmonary disease

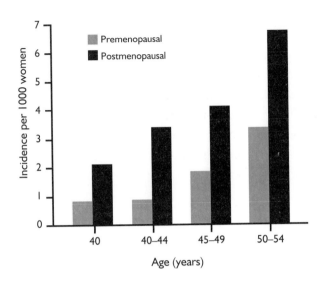

Figure 6.3

Incidence of cardiovascular disease in premenopausal and postmenopausal women. Reproduced from reference 4 with permission

There are many factors which may contribute to an increased risk of CHD (Table 6.1). Some risk factors may be modified or altered by hormone therapy, and others by a change in lifestyle.

Table 6.1   Risk factors for cardiovascular disease

Family history

Smoking

Elevated blood cholesterol and triglycerides

High blood pressure

Increased level of clotting factors

Diabetes

Obesity

Lack of exercise

6.3 Smoking

Smoking has long been known to be a principal risk factor for CHD, and is related to the length of time and the number of cigarettes smoked per day. In recent years, smoking rates have significantly declined, but have done so less in women, and particularly in younger women (Figure 6.4)[5]. In addition, smoking has a strong multiplicative effect on risk with other factors such as diabetes and hypertension[2].

6.4 Obesity and body fat distribution

The body mass index (BMI) is the easiest way of assessing obesity, and is a measure of weight adjusted for height. BMI equals weight (kg)/height (m)^2 (see Appendix). There is an increase in cardiac risk associated with a body mass index above 25. The

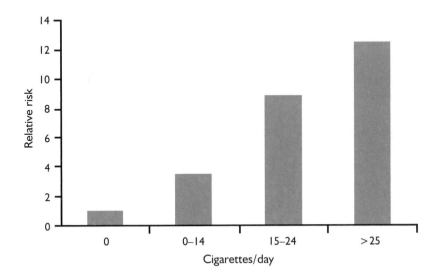

Figure 6.4

Relationship between number of cigarettes smoked and risk of myocardial infarction in women below the age of 55. Reproduced from reference 5 with permission

distribution of body fat is also related to the ocurrence of CHD, and has been shown to be a more important risk factor than obesity *per se* in women. Central (android) fat distribution – where fat accumulates around the trunk and abdominal cavity – is associated with an adverse lipid profile (particularly hypertriglyceridemia and low levels of high-density lipoprotein (HDL)), insulin resistance and increased risk of CHD. In contrast, lower-body (gynoid) fat distribution – where fat accumulates particularly around the hips, thighs and buttocks – does not appear to be related to increased risk of CHD[6].

6.5 Lipids

The postmenopausal decline in estrogen results in several biochemical changes which can promote cardiovascular disease. Notable among these is an increase in blood cholesterol levels. There are two main types of cholesterol: HDL and low-density lipoprotein (LDL) cholesterol. HDL encourages the uptake of cholesterol to the liver, where it is metabolized. The effect of HDL, therefore, is favorable. LDL cholesterol, however, has an unfavorable effect as it transfers cholesterol to the walls of the arteries, leading to atherosclerosis (Figure 6.5). The menopause is associated with an increase in total cholesterol of about 20%, of LDL by about 30%, and a decrease in HDL of up to 25%. In addition, the level of triglycerides may increase by 10–15%, which is a further unfavorable factor[7]. *The relative risk of CHD increases by 37% in women for each 1 mmol/l increase in plasma triglyceride concentration.*

6.6 Diabetes

Diabetes is a particular risk factor for cardiovascular disease in women, and increases the risk of cardiac mortality by more than double that of men[8]. Smoking compounds this risk, and with 15 or more cigarettes a day it is more than seven times greater[9].

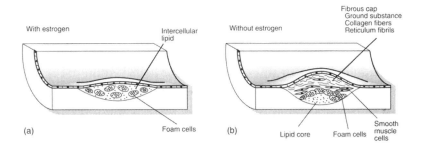

Figure 6.5

Representation of atheromatous coronary vessels in the presence of estrogen (a) and in the estrogen-deficient state (b). Reproduced from Collins P, Beale CM. *The Cardioprotective Role of HT: a Clinical Update.* Carnforth, UK: Parthenon Publishing, 1996

6.7   Potential cardioprotective effects of HT

The effects of HT on the risk factors for cardiovascular disease have been extensively researched over many years, and have indicated that potential cardioprotective effects could be the result of both metabolic and of direct effects on the arterial walls[10] (Table 6.2):

- HT reduces the levels of total cholesterol by up to 10% irrespective of the type or route of administration (Figure 6.6)[11]

- Oral estrogen lowers LDL. There is a smaller reduction in LDL with transdermal estrogen

- Oral estrogen increases HDL. There is less effect on HDL with transdermal estrogen

- Oral estrogen tends to increase triglycerides which is unfavorable. Estrogen given by non-oral routes tends to cause a decrease in triglyceride (Figure 6.7)[11]

Table 6.2 Metabolic changes with different HT preparations and routes of administration. Reproduced from reference 12 with permission

	Estrogen component				Progestogen component	
	Oral CEE	Oral estradiol (2 mg)	Oral estradiol (1 mg)	Estradiol (transdermal)	Oral MPA	Oral norethisterone
Lipids						
Triglyceride	↑↑	↑	↑/→	→	↓	↓
HDL cholesterol	↑↑	↑↑	↑	→	↓	↓
LDL cholesterol	↓↓	↓↓	↓	→	→	→
Coagulation						
Factor VII		↑↑	↑↑	↑	↓	↓
C-reactive protein	↑↑	↑	→	ND/→	ND	↓

CEE, conjugated equine estrogen; MPA, medroxyprogesterone acetate; ND, not done

- Estrogen causes the release of chemicals from the arterial walls, such as nitric oxide, which encourages vasodilatation, i.e. relaxation of the blood vessels, which become wider, allowing blood to flow more easily

- Estrogen given by a non-oral route reduces the levels of clotting factors and therefore decreases the potential for thrombosis

- Estrogen reduces the levels of homocysteine in the blood. Homocysteine is an amino acid, an excess of which contributes to atherosclerosis. High homocysteine levels are associated with low levels of vitamin B_6 and folic acid, and it has been suggested that dietary supplementation may be protective

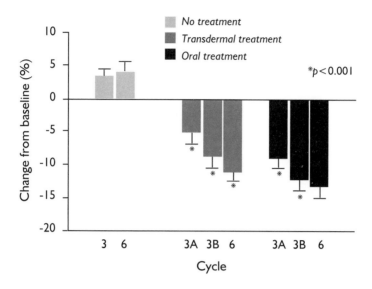

Figure 6.6

Effect of HT on total cholesterol. Transdermal treatment, estradiol and norethisterone acetate; oral treatment, conjugated equine estrogens and levonorgestrel; 3A, estrogen alone; 3B, combined therapy; 6, combined therapy. Reproduced from reference 11 with permission

- Estrogen does not increase blood pressure and may reduce it in hypertensive women. Hypertension is not a contra-indication to HT, which may complement the effects of antihypertensive therapy

- Estrogen reduces exercise-induced myocardial ischemia in postmenopausal women with established CHD[13]

6.8   Does the addition of progestogen modify the possible beneficial effects of estrogen?

Most of the studies relating to estrogen and cardiovascular disease have involved women who have used unopposed conjugated equine estrogens. Progestogens are needed to protect the

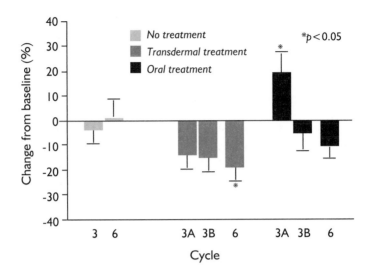

Figure 6.7

Effect of HT on triglyceride levels. Transdermal treatment, estradiol and norethisterone acetate; oral treatment, conjugated equine estrogens and levonorgestrel; 3A, estrogen alone; 3B, combined therapy; 6, combined therapy. Reproduced from reference 11 with permission

endometrium, and since they are known to counteract some of the biochemical and physiological effects of estrogen, there have been concerns that they would reduce or eliminate some cardio-protective effects. This is one reason why there are relatively fewer prescriptions for combined therapy in the USA compared to Europe, and many more women have unopposed estrogen. Information about the effect of progestogen addition is relatively sparse, and what there is, is confusing. Animal studies have shown that medroxyprogesterone acetate (MPA) reduces the ability of estrogen to inhibit atherosclerosis, whereas progesterone does not[14] (Figure 6.8). Further recent data, however, from the WELL-HART research group show that, in women with a mean age of 63.5 years and established coronary artery atherosclerosis, 17β-estradiol either alone or with sequentially administered MPA had no significant effect on the progression of atherosclerosis[15]. However, two studies into the incidence of heart attacks in women using estrogen alone or in combination with different progestogens, showed that the risk was reduced more than with unopposed estrogen[1,16].

It is well recognized that different progestogens have different metabolic effects and this may be relevant for the comparison of different HT regimens in their effect on cardiovascular disease risk. In the future, systemic exposure to progestogens may be reduced by using a locally acting intrauterine device (such as Mirena®), which releases progestogen into the endometrial cavity with minimal spill into the circulation[17].

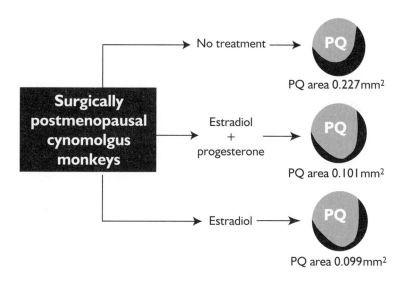

Figure 6.8

Inhibition of atherosclerosis by estradiol in ovariectomized monkeys. PQ, plaque (black area). Adapted from reference 14 with permission

6.9 Recent research suggests that HT might have an initial negative effect in women with established cardiovascular disease

The first randomized trial to assess the cardioprotective effects of estrogen in women with pre-existing cardiovascular disease was the HERS study (Heart and Estrogen/progestin Replacement Study)[18]. This showed that while estrogen lowered LDL cholesterol and raised HDL cholesterol, it did not prevent heart disease. In fact, there was a small increase in coronary deaths in the first year of treatment, and only a small fall in death rate in subsequent years. However, the death rate did fall by 33% by years 4 and 5 of the trial. The findings of the HERS trial provoked anxious debate amongst physicians, who pointed to flaws in the methodology of the study. The mean age of the women was 67 years, and they all received conjugated equine estrogens (CEE) 0.625 mg, together with MPA 5 mg daily, a combination that has not previously been studied, and one which provides a relatively higher dose of estrogen than would usually be given to women of this age. Also the trial design did not include an estrogen-only group.

Other lines of research have, however, indicated that estrogen could be useful in secondary prevention after a heart attack, or in the presence of coronary disease. It shows a beneficial effect on coronary oxygen lack brought on by exercise, and has a relaxant effect on atherosclerotic coronary arteries[13,19]. Following the HERS and the more recent WHI study[20], most physicians are reluctant to prescribe HT for women with existing cardiovascular disease. But, a recent pilot study of 100 postmenopausal women who were between 48 hours and 28 days following an acute myocardial infarction, found a lower death rate and fewer further admissions to hospital in those who were given low-dose HT with oral estradiol 1 mg daily and norethisterone acetate 0.5 mg daily, compared to those receiving a placebo[21].

6.10   Women's Health Initiative study suggests increase in heart disease with HT

The largest prospective study of the effects of hormone therapy in postmenopausal women has been the US Women's Health Initiative (WHI) study[20]. Briefly, the study included more than 16 000 healthy postmenopausal women aged 50–79 years who were randomized to receive either CEE 0.625 mg with MPA 2.5 mg daily, or a placebo. The study was planned to run for 8.5 years but was stopped after 5.2 years in mid-2002, because women in the treatment group had an increased incidence of breast cancer, and because an overall measure suggested that the treatment was causing more harm than good. The other major concerns were an increase in coronary heart disease, with a hazard ratio (HR) of 1.29 (95% confidence interval (CI) 1.02–1.63), an increase in stroke, HR 1.41 (95% CI 1.07–1.85) and pulmonary embolism, HR 2.13 (95% CI 1.39–3.25).

Regrettably, the media chose to highlight these findings in percentage terms of relative risk, such that the increase in breast cancer was 26%, coronary heart disease 29%, stroke 41% and pulmonary embolism 213%. However, when the figures are given as absolute risk, for 10 000 women taking HT each year, the findings represent an extra eight cases of breast cancer, seven heart attacks, eight strokes and eight pulmonary embolisms. These figures put the risks into a more appropriate and understandable perspective. Nevertheless, the increased risk of cardiovascular disease is surprising and disappointing. It is not clear whether these findings can be extrapolated to all other combinations of estrogen and progestogen, and other routes of administration. However, it is well established that progestogens have different metabolic effects, and non-oral routes of hormone delivery also produce different changes to the oral route, so it would be inappropriate to extrapolate to all forms of hormone therapy.

The WHI study also has an estrogen-only arm for women who have had a hysterectomy, which has not been stopped, implying that it is the MPA that is causing the harmful effects. This part of the study may possibly demonstrate some beneficial effects. One of the main concerns about the relevance of the HERS and WHI studies is that the women had an average age of around 65 years, and were given a relatively high dose of combined HT with the intention of establishing if there was any benefit particularly for cardiovascular disease, either in women with or without pre-existing evidence of cardiovascular problems. In clinical practice, most women are given HT at a much younger age in order to relieve menopausal symptoms, and few will be starting HT in their mid-60s as in these studies. It is therefore difficult to establish the implications of these study results for the majority of women who may be seeking or are prescribed HT for the benefits of improved quality of life. At present, it would seem reasonable to offer advice as suggested below.

6.11   Advice to women concerning HT and the heart

- Women should not be given any regimen of continuous combined HT solely for the prevention of cardiovascular disease, for which other well-proven measures such as lipid-lowering agents, antihypertensive therapy and lifestyle factors would be more appropriate

- Women who are already taking the same combination of hormones as used in the HERS and WHI studies (CEE and MPA) should be advised of the findings of these studies so that they can decide if they wish to continue, stop or change to another regimen. They should also be advised that there are no data on the long-term safety of any other regimen

- At present, unopposed estrogen may seem to be a safer option, but this is less suitable for those who have not had a hysterectomy (see also Section 8.7). Such women may be reassured that concerns about cardiovascular risk from the WHI study do not apply to unopposed estrogen, for which the effects are awaited from continuation of this arm of the study

- For most women, the maintenance of a healthy lifestyle with attention to diet, not smoking, weight and exercise will be of far greater value in preventing cardiovascular disease than hormone therapy

6.12 Is raloxifene a suitable alternative to HT?

The SERM raloxifene (see Section 2.7) has favorable effects on LDL cholesterol and other risk factors for CHD[22,23] and improves vascular endothelial function in postmenopausal women[24]. The RUTH trial (Raloxifene Use for The Heart)[25] is a 5-year international prospective study, involving 10 101 post-menopausal women with existing coronary disease, which aims to assess the effects of raloxifene on several cardiovascular disease end-points. Because raloxifene does not stimulate the endometrium, it is not necessary to use additional progestogen. The trial will report in 2004 and should help to elucidate the role of SERMs in secondary prevention. However, the MORE study[26] of 7705 postmenopausal women with osteoporosis has shown that raloxifene therapy for 4 years did not significantly affect the risk of cardiovascular events overall, but analysis of those with increased risk of CVD found a reduction of events such as myocardial infarction, angina, stroke and transient ischemic attacks that was significant (RR = 0.60; 95% CI 0.38–0.95).

6.13 The relationship between HT in menopausal women and stroke is unclear

While combined oral contraceptives may increase a younger woman's risk of stroke[27,28], the relationship between HT in menopausal women and stroke remains unclear.

Table 6.3   Risk of stroke. Data from reference 29

Age (years)	Excess absolute risk per 10 000 women per year
50–59	4
60–69	9
70–79	13

Few studies have ever shown any significant benefit from HT on the risk of stroke, but most have failed to differentiate between the different types of stroke or the wide variety of potential risk factors.

The HERS investigators found no increase in stroke but WHI has found an increased risk of ischemic but not of hemorrhagic stroke with the particular continuous combined estrogen and progestogen regimen (CEE 0.625 mg and MPA 2.5 mg daily)[29]. The risk increased with age (Table 6.3).

At age 50 years, a woman faces an estimated 20% probability of developing a stroke within her lifetime and an 8% probability of dying from a stroke[30]. The two major types of stroke are infarction (85%) and hemorrhagic (10%). For infarction, ischemic injury occurs as a direct consequence of diminished blood flow. For hemorrhagic, vascular rupture into the subarachnoid space or brain tissue causes neuronal death mainly through tissue compression and secondary vasospasm. Both infarction and hemorrhage are primarily diseases of the arterial system and venous strokes are rare[31]. In Western countries, stroke is the third leading cause of death, exceeded only by ischemic heart disease and cancer.

References

1. Grodstein F, Stampfer MJ, Manson JE, et al. Postmenopausal estrogen and progestin use and the risk of cardiovascular disease. *N Engl J Med* 1996;335:453–61

2. Lloyd GW, Jackson G. Pre-menopausal risk factors for coronary artery disease. *J Br Menop Soc* 2002;8:108–11

3. Mosca L, Jones WK, King KB, et al. Awareness, perception, and knowledge of heart disease risk and prevention among women in the United States. American Heart Association Women's Heart Disease and Stroke Campaign Task Force. *Arch Fam Med* 2000;9:506–15

4. Gordon T, Kannel WB, Hjortland MC, et al. Menopause and coronary heart disease: the Framingham study. *Ann Intern Med* 1978;89:157–61

5. Dunn NR, Faragher B, Thorogood M, et al. Risk of myocardial infarction in young female smokers. *Heart* 1999;82:581–3

6. Stevenson JC. HT and cardiovascular disease. In Barlow DH, ed. *Essentials of HT and the Menopause*. London: Science Press Limited, 2001

7. Stevenson JC, Crook D, Godsland IF. Influence of age and menopause on serum lipids and lipoproteins in healthy women. *Atherosclerosis* 1993;98:83–90

8. Lerner D, Kannel W. Patterns of coronary heart disease morbidity and mortality in the sexes: a 26 year follow up of the Framingham population. *Am Heart J* 1986;111:383–90

9. Al-Delaimy WK, Manson JE, Solomon CG, et al. Smoking and risk of coronary heart disease among women with Type II diabetes mellitus. *Arch Intern Med* 2002;162:273–9

10. Stevenson JC. Metabolic effects of the menopause and oestrogen replacement. *Baillière's Clin Obstet Gynaecol* 1996;10:449–67

11. Crook D, Stevenson JC. Effects of estrogens on serum lipids and lipoproteins. In Ahlquist J, Wass J, eds. *Endocrine Replacement Therapy: New Approaches*. London: Royal College of Physicians, 1996

12. Bain C, Lumsden MA, Sattar N, Greer I. *The Menopause in Practice*. London: RSM Press Limited, 2003

13. Rosano GM, Sarrel PM, Poole-Wilson PA, *et al*. Beneficial effect of estrogen on exercise-induced myocardial ischaemia in women with coronary artery disease. *Lancet* 1993;342:133-6

14. Adams MR, Kaplan JR, Manuck SB, *et al*. Inhibition of coronary artery atherosclerosis by 17-β estradiol in ovariectomised monkeys: lack of an effect of added progesterone. *Arteriosclerosis* 1990;10:1051–7

15. Hadis HN, Mack WJ, Azen SP, *et al*. Hormone therapy and the progression of coronary artery atherosclerosis in post-menopausal women. *N Engl J Med* 2003;349:535–45

16. Falkeborn M, Persson I, Adami HO, *et al*. The risk of acute myocardial infarction after oestrogen and oestrogen/progestogen replacement. *Br J Obstet Gynaecol* 1992;99:821–8

17. Riphagen FE. Intrauterine application of progestins in hormone replacement therapy. *Climacteric* 2000;3:199–211

18. Hulley ST, Grady D, Bush T, *et al*. For the Heart and Estrogen/Progestin Replacement Study (HERS) Research Group. Randomized trial of estrogen plus progestin for secondary prevention of coronary heart disease in postmenopausal women. *J Am Med Assoc* 1998;280:605–13

19. Williams JK, Adams MR, Klopfenstein S. Estrogen modulates responses of atherosclerotic coronary arteries. *Circulation* 1990;81:1680

20. Writing Group for the Women's Health Initiative Investigators. Risks and benefits of estrogen plus progestin in healthy postmenopausal women. *J Am Med Assoc* 2002;288:321–33

21. Stevenson JC, Lees B, Mister R, *et al.* The Womens Hormone Intervention Secondary Prevention (WHISP) pilot study. 10th World Congress on the Menopause, Berlin. *Climacteric* 2002;5(Suppl 1):55 abstr F-04-03

22. Walsh BW, Kuller LH, Wild RA, *et al.* Effects of raloxifene on serum lipids and coagulation factors in healthy postmenopausal women. *J Am Med Assoc* 1998;279:1445–51

23. Walsh BW, Paul S, Wild RA, *et al.* The effects of hormone replacement therapy and raloxifene on C-reactive protein and homocysteine in healthy postmenopausal women: a randomised, controlled trial. *J Clin Endocrinol Metab* 2000;85:214–18

24. Saitta A, Altavilla D, Cucinotta D, *et al.* Randomized, double-blind, placebo controlled study on the effects of raloxifene and hormone replacement therapy on plasma nitric oxide concentrations, endothelin-1 levels and endothelium-dependent vasodilatation in postmenopausal women. *Arterioscler Thromb Vasc Biol* 2001;21:1512–19

25. Mosca L, Barrett-Connor E, Wenger NK, *et al.* Design and methods of the Raloxifene Use for The Heart (RUTH) study. *Am J Cardiol* 2001;88:392–5

26. Barrett-Connor E, Grady D, Sashegyi A, *et al.* Raloxifene and cardiovascular events in osteoporotic postmenopausal women.

Four-year results from the MORE (Multiple Outcomes of Raloxifene Evaluation) randomized trial. *J Am Med Assoc* 2002;287:847–57

27. Vessey M, Painter R, Yeates D. Mortality in relation to oral contraceptive use and cigarette smoking. *Lancet* 2003;362:185–91

28. WHO Collaborative Study of Cardiovascular Disease and Steroid Contraception. Hemorrhagic stroke, overall stroke risk and combined oral contraceptives: results of an international, multi-centre, case–control study. *Lancet* 1996;348:505–10

29. Wassertheil-Smoller S, Hendrix SL, Limacher M, *et al*. Effect of estrogen plus progestin on stroke in postmenopausal women: the Women's Health Initiative: a randomized trial. *J Am Med Assoc* 2003;289:2673–84

30. Grady D, Rubin SM, Petitti DB, *et al*. Hormone therapy to prevent disease and prolong life in postmenopausal women. *Ann Intern Med* 1992;117:1016–37

31. Henderson VW. *Hormone Therapy and the Brain*. Carnforth, UK: Parthenon Publishing, 2000

Chapter 7

HT and the brain

7.1 Estrogen modifies many aspects of brain activity

Estrogen exerts significant effects on the brain. It affects brain development in the fetus, causing structural changes in the female brain which differentiate it from the male. It facilitates the growth of nerve cells and their interconnections. Estrogen modifies the synthesis and metabolism of several neurotransmitters. These are chemicals released by brain cells, which stimulate reactions in adjacent cells, and which play a pivotal role in intercellular communication. Estrogen influences the brain region called the hypothalamus, where the centers for control of body temperature are located. Reduced levels of estrogen modify the effects of neurotransmitters in the hypothalamus, causing a temporary impairment of its thermoregulatory activity, which is the likely cause of hot flushes and sweats[1].

Estrogen receptors have been found in numerous areas of the brain, including those involved in emotion[2]. Decreases in neurotransmitters in these areas are known to contribute to depression, and estrogen modifies their activity towards mood enhancement. Table 7.1 illustrates the multiple systems on which estrogen acts, and it can be seen that, in each case, the change caused by estrogen on neurotransmitter levels opposes the change caused by depression. The antidepressant paroxetine [Prozac®] acts by increasing the concentration of the neurotransmitter serotonin, and endorphins are 'feel good' chemicals released in response to physical exercise and other stimuli. Estrogen increases the levels of both of them, along with other important chemicals known to enhance mood. It would appear then that estrogen is an important natural antidepressant.

7.2 The contribution of menopausal estrogen decline to depression is a matter of some controversy

It would seem logical, therefore, that the menopausal reduction in estrogen should predispose women to depression at this stage in their lives, and that HT should have a beneficial effect. Depression is more common in women than in men, and this applies across all cultures, races and socioeconomic groupings, and at all ages after puberty. Depression is currently ranked by

Table 7.1 Changes in neurotransmitters caused by estrogen and depression. Modified from reference 3

Changes caused by estrogen	Changes caused by depression
• Serotonin ↓	• Serotonin ↑
• Noradrenaline ↓	• Noradrenaline ↑
• Dopamine ↓↑	• Dopamine ↑↓
• Monoamine oxidase ↑	• Monoamine oxidase ↓
• γ-aminobutyric acid ↓	• γ-aminobutyric acid ↑
• Endorphin ↓	• Endorphin ↑
• β-adrenergic receptors ↑	• β-adrenergic receptors ↓

Table 7.2   Factors which contribute to depressed mood at the menopause

Psychosocial factors	Personal attributes
• Worry about family	• Low self-esteem
• Traditional gender role	• Emotional dependency
• Care of elderly parents	• External locus of control (belief that
• Aging of partner	factors 'out there' have more influence
• Separation/divorce	on your life than you do)
• Lack of good social network	• Low expectations
• Monotonous job with no control	• Negative attitude to the menopause
• Unemployment	• Negative attitude to aging
	• Inappropriate learned coping mechanisms
Health status	• Low educational attainment
• Poor physical health	
• Menopausal symptoms	

the World Health Organization as the world's fourth most devastating disease.

However, the evidence for a decrease in mental health at the menopause is conflicting. As stated in Chapter 4, women attending menopause clinics frequently report psychological symptoms. Some studies have reported that 20% of menopausal women experience depressed mood[4,5], while others have concluded that the menopause does not have a significant effect on a variety of common psychiatric symptoms[6].

There is also uncertainty about whether estrogen deficiency is causative in those women who do report psychological disturbance at the menopause. It is difficult to disentangle the effects of low estrogen from the numerous other factors that have been shown to predict depression in menopausal women. These are summarized in Table 7.2, and it is not surprising that researchers disagree about the extent to which changing hormonal patterns are influential. Neither have the research methodologies used in this field always been sufficiently rigorous to provide definitive answers, nor is there agreement as to the best means of measuring psychological changes. The distinction between clinical depression and lowered mood has not always been made. These complications make it difficult to evaluate and compare the research in this field.

7.3   HT elevates mood in menopausal women

Despite the above concerns, a number of clinical studies suggest that estrogen replacement both improves mood and brings an increased sense of well-being in menopausal women, including those who do not report psychological symptoms[2,7]. It has also been shown to alleviate symptoms such as irritability, anxiety, lack of self-confidence and depression. This was also true of women who did not suffer from hot flushes, suggesting a direct effect of estrogen on mental status rather than just through symptom relief[8].

Clear evidence has emerged that depression is more likely to result from fluctuating, rather than low blood estrogen[9]. No differences have been found between the estrogen levels of depressed and asymptomatic women, suggesting that absolute levels are not the key to depression. Women who experience sudden drops in estrogen following removal of their ovaries are more liable to depression, and replacement estrogen is used to prevent psychiatric morbidity in this situation[10,11]. A long perimenopausal stage is associated with an increased incidence of depression, and psychological symptoms are more common in the 45–49-year age group, i.e. at the time when estrogen profiles are likely to be erratic[12]. Women who report depression at the menopause are more likely to have a history of premenstrual syndrome and postnatal depression, again times when hormone levels fluctuate. Estrogen therapy is effective in these women. In this connection it is interesting that depression is rare in the third trimester of pregnancy, when estrogen levels are very high.

Severe or clinical depression in postmenopausal women does not respond to the doses of estrogen used in HT, and such women should have primary treatment with conventional anti-depressants. However, in perimenopausal women there is evidence that estrogen is helpful. One randomized, controlled study reported remission of depression in 68% of perimenopausal women treated with transdermal estradiol 100 µg daily compared to 20% improvement with placebo ($p = 0.001$)[13].

The HERS trial[14] found that hormone therapy had a mixed effect on the quality of life among older women depending on the presence of menopausal symptoms. Women with hot flushes who had hormone therapy had a significant improvement in mental health and fewer depressive symptoms during follow-up, compared with those assigned to the placebo. Hormone therapy is not expected to improve the quality of life or mental state of women who are asymptomatic, and recent newspaper headlines that hormone therapy was no better than placebo in improving quality of life from the WHI study[15], ignore the fact that the women in this study were selected because they were asympto-matic. This is analogous to giving aspirin to a woman who does not have a headache and being surprised that it did not make her feel any different!

Severe depression does not respond to the doses of estrogen used in HT. One groundbreaking study showed that very high doses of estrogen had significant antidepressant effects in severely depressed women who had not responded to conventional treatment.

In summary, women who take HT primarily to help with the physical symptoms of the menopause will experience the bonus of the 'mental tonic' provided by estrogen, while those who experience psychological symptoms may well experience an improvement on HT. There is a difference between depressed mood and clinical depression, but if other menopausal symptoms are present the chances of successful treatment with hormone therapy are greater, and it is certainly worth trying HT in such women, assuming there is no contraindication. Depression that is not associated with menopausal symptoms, particularly in women who are postmenopausal, is less likely to respond to hormone therapy and conventional antidepressants should be considered.

7.4   Estrogen improves cognitive function

Generally, there is little difference between men and women in overall cognitive performance, although on average men perform better in tests of visual-spacial function, and women are usually better at verbal tests. There is considerable evidence that sex hormones modulate various aspects of cognitive function, and in healthy women, cognitive abilities vary with the phases of the menstrual cycle, with improved fine motor and articulatory skills and improved memory performance during the high estrogen and low progestogen phase of the cycle[16]. The effects of estrogen were also demonstrated in women randomized to receive estrogen replacement or placebo following hysterectomy and removal of both ovaries (Figure 7.1).

Randomized trials have demonstrated that the women who are likely to find an improvement in cognitive function with hormone therapy are those who are also experiencing menopausal symptoms, and little obvious benefit for women without associated symptoms. However, one study of over 2000 healthy elderly women reported that current users of HT performed much better than never users on verbal fluency tasks, whereas there was no difference in overall cognitive ability[17].

7.5   HT may delay the onset of Alzheimer's disease

Alzheimer's disease (AD) is the commonest form of dementia, and involves the loss of mental capacity severe enough to interfere significantly with the performance of everyday

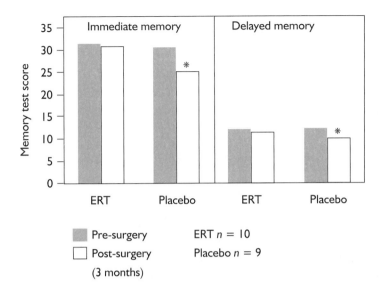

Figure 7.1

The protective effect of estrogen on immediate and delayed verbal memory in surgically menopausal women. *$p < 0.05$; ERT, estrogen replacement therapy. Adapted with permission from reference 16

activities. Dementia affects mainly the elderly and the prevalence doubles every 5 years after the age of 60[18], rising to 47% of those over the age of 85 years. Women are more genetically predisposed to suffer from AD than men[19] (Figure 7.2). Given the projected figures for the number of women who will survive into their 80s (Table 1.2), late-onset AD is set to become a major public health issue.

Alzheimer's disease progresses slowly and insidiously. The first symptom is usually a reduced facility for remembering recent events or new information, and this is followed by the deterioration of other cognitive abilities, such as low attention span, forgetting the names of everyday things, failure to recognize family members, and loss of reasoning power. Sometimes these cognitive changes are associated with a change in personality, e.g. apathy, depression and delusional thinking.

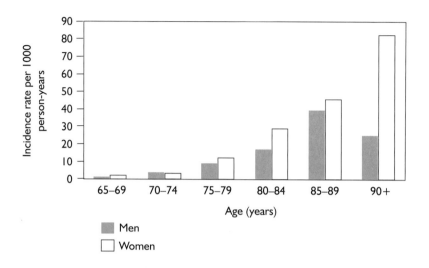

Figure 7.2

Comparison of the incidence of Alzheimer's disease in men and women. Adapted with permission from Andersen K, Launer LJ, Dewey ME, *et al.* Gender differences in the incidence of AD and vascular dementia: the EURODEM Studies. EURODEM Incidence Research Group. *Neurology* 1999;53:1992–7

Alzheimer's disease results from pathological changes in the nerve cells in key areas of the brain, particularly in those regions that influence cognitive processes. The nerve cells gradually lose many of their connections with neighboring cells, and develop abnormal intracellular proteins. The surrounding tissue develops inflammatory plaques of distorted nerve cell processes containing an abnormal protein, amyloid, which is also present in the cerebral blood vessels.

There is accumulating clinical evidence from prospective trials that estrogen may both delay or prevent the onset of AD. One study carried out in the Leisure World retirement community in California showed that estrogen users were 35% less likely to develop AD, and that the risk reduction was greatest in those who had used it for longest or at higher doses[20]. Research in several other centers has borne out these findings[21-23]. Estrogen use decreased the risk by about 50%, and raised the age at which AD was first diagnosed. However, it has to be said that not all studies have demonstrated a protective effect of estrogen[24] and more research is needed to confirm the findings.

A few studies have indicated that estrogen replacement therapy may ameliorate the symptoms of established disease, with treated women performing better on several measures of cognitive ability[25]. However, three other randomized, double-blind, placebo-controlled trials have been less optimistic. In these trials, 97, 50 and 40 subjects with mild to moderate AD took conjugated equine estrogens for 12, 3 and 4 months, respectively. There were no beneficial effects on cognition, mood or functional outcomes in these patients[26]. In contrast, a more recent study reported a significant treatment benefit after just 4 weeks of estradiol patches[27]. So it is not clear whether estrogen does provide benefit for patients with established AD and certainly it will not seem to be justified to give HT just for this purpose, but there may well be some benefit in preventing the onset of the disease.

There is an attractive theory that there is a 'window of opportunity' during which the pathological disease processes involved in the development of AD, and possibly coronary artery disease, may be delayed if estrogen therapy is commenced. However, if treatment is started after the pathological process has commenced, there is less likelihood of having any effect on the disease process.

7.6 Mechanisms by which HT may help in Alzheimer's disease

There are several mechanisms whereby estrogen may reduce the risk of AD and these are summarized in Table 7.3. Of particular significance is its effect on the neurotransmitter system that

Table 7.3   Effects of estrogen that may reduce the risk of Alzheimer's disease

- Stimulates numerous factors that promote the growth of nerve cells and their interconnections

- Prevents formation of amyloid protein, which is the characteristic of Alzheimer's disease, and increases the breakdown of existing amyloid

- Reduces inflammation

- Protects against brain cell apoptosis (programmed cell death)

- Increases blood flow to the brain

involves acetylcholine. This neurotransmitter has an important role in cognitive processes. It is found in those parts of the brain that are particularly susceptible to the pathological cell changes that characterize AD. Alzheimer patients have been shown to have few receptors for acetylcholine[28], and therapy that increases brain levels of acetylcholine improves their cognitive abilities. This is more marked if the patient also receives estrogen[29]. Estrogen therapy has been shown to restore acetylcholine receptors in rats whose ovaries were removed, and long-term use of hormone therapy in postmenopausal women protects against loss of responsiveness to acetylcholine[28].

The research into the protective effects of estrogen in preventing AD is not yet at the stage where recommendations for treatment can be given. However, future research may indicate that this could be another reason for longer-term use of hormone therapy in postmenopausal women.

References

1.   Meldrum DK, De Fazio J, Erlik Y, et al. Pituitary hormones during the menopausal hot flush. *Obstet Gynecol* 1984;64:752–62

2. Sherwin B. Impact of the changing hormonal milieu on psychological functioning. In Lobo RA, ed. *Treatment of the Postmenopausal Woman: Basic and Clinical Aspects*. New York: Raven Press, 1994:119–27

3. Archer JS. Depression, oestrogen and neurotransmitters in postmenopause. In Studd J, ed. *The Management of the Menopause: The Millennium Review 2000*. Carnforth, UK: Parthenon Publishing, 2000:129–38

4. Holte A. Influence of natural menopause on health complaints: a prospective study of healthy Norwegian women. *Maturitas* 1992;14:127–41

5. Kaufert P, Gilbert P, Tate R. The Manitoba project: a re-examination of the link between menopause and depression. *Maturitas* 1992;14:143–55

6. Ballinger CB. Psychiatric aspects of the menopause. *Br J Psychiatr* 1990;56:73–87

7. Ditkoff EC, Crary WG, Cristo M, Lobo RA. Estrogen improves psychological functioning in asymptomatic postmenopausal women. *Obstet Gynecol* 1991;78:991–5

8. Campbell S, Whitehead M. Oestrogen therapy and the menopausal syndrome. *Clin Obstet Gynaecol* 1977;1:31–47

9. Sherwin BB. Hormones, mood and cognitive functioning in post-menopausal women. *Obstet Gynecol* 1996;87:20–6

10. Khastgir G, Studd J. Hysterectomy, ovarian failure and depression. *Menopause* 1998;5:113–22

11. Vliet EL, Davis VLH. New perspectives on the relationship of hormone changes to affective disorders in the perimenopause. *NAACOGS Clin Issu Perinat Women's Health Nurs* 1991;2:453–71

12. Studd JWW, Panay N. Estrogens in the treatment of climacteric depression, premenstrual depression, postnatal depression and chronic fatigue syndrome. In Wren BG, ed. *Progress in the Management of the Menopause*. Carnforth, UK: Parthenon Publishing, 1996:385–92

13. Soares CN, Almeida OP, Joffe H, Cohen LS. Efficacy of oestradiol for the treatment of depressive disorders in peri-menopausal women; a double-blind, randomised, placebo-controlled trial. *Arch Gen Psychiatr* 2001;58:529–34

14. Hlatky MA, Boothroyd D, Vittinghoff E, Sharp P, Whooley MA. Quality of life and depressive symptoms in postmenopausal women after receiving hormone therapy; results from the Heart and Estrogen/progestin Replacement Study (HERS) Trial. *J Am Med Assoc* 2002;287:591–7

15. Hayes J, Ockene JK, Brunner RL, *et al*. Effects of estrogen plus progestin on health-related quality of life. *N Engl J Med* 2003;348:1–15

16. Phillips SM, Sherwin BB. Effects of estrogen on memory function in surgically menopausal women. *Psychoneuroendocrinology* 1992;17:485–95

17. Grodstein F, Chen J, Pollen DA, *et al*. Postmenopausal hormone therapy and cognitive function in healthy older women. *J Am Geriatr Soc* 2000;48:746–52

18. Katzman R. Education and the prevalence of dementia and Alzheimer's disease. *Neurology* 1993;43:13–20

19. Payami H, Zareparsi S, Montee KR, *et al*. Gender difference in apolipoprotein E-associated risk for familial Alzheimer disease: a possible clue to the higher incidence of Alzheimer's disease in women. *Am J Hum Genet* 1996;58:803–11

20. Paganini-Hill A, Henderson VW. Estrogen replacement therapy and risk of Alzheimer disease. *Arch Intern Med* 1996;156:2213–17

21. Tang M-X, Jacobs D, Stern Y, *et al*. Effect of oestrogen during menopause on risk and age at onset of Alzheimer's disease. *Lancet* 1996;348:429–32

22. Kawas C, Resnick S, Morrison A, *et al*. A prospective study of estrogen replacement therapy and the risk of developing Alzheimer's disease; the Baltimore Longitudinal Study of Aging. *Neurology* 1997;48:1517–21

23. Waring SC, Rocca WA, Petersen RC, Kokemen E. Postmenopausal estrogen replacement therapy and the risk of developing Alzheimer's disease; a population-based study in Rochester, Minesota. *Neurology* 1997;48(Suppl 2): abstr A729

24. Brenner DE, Kukall WA, Stergachis A, *et al*. Postmenopausal estrogen replacement therapy and the risk of Alzheimer's disease: a population-based case-controlled study. *Am J Epidemiol* 1994;140:262–7

25. Henderson VW. Estrogen replacement therapy for the prevention and treatment of Alzheimer's disease. *CNS Drugs* 1997;8:343–51

26. Wang PN, Liao SQ, Liu RS, *et al*. The effects of estrogen on cognition, mood, and verbal blood flow in Alzheimer's disease: a controlled study. *Neurology* 2000;54:2061–6

27. Asthana S, Baker LD, Craft S, *et al*. High-dose estradiol improves cognition for women with Alzheimer's disease: results of a randomised study. *Neurology* 2001;57:605–12

28. Muire JL. Acetylcholine, aging and Alzheimer's disease. *Pharmacol Biochem Behav* 1997;56:687–96

29. Schneider LS, Farlow MR, Henderson VW, *et al.* Effects of estrogen replacement therapy on response to tacrine in patients with Alzheimer's disease. *Neurology* 1996;46:1580–4

See also:

Hormone replacement therapy in climacteric aging brain. International Menopause Society Expert Workshop, Pisa, March 15–18, 2003. *Climacteric* 2003;6:186–203

Chapter 8

Obstacles to HT use

8.1 Few women start HT or continue treatment beyond 12 months

It is estimated that only 20% of women in the USA have ever used HT, and that less than 8% are still on therapy after 1 year[1]. The recent British Million Women Study[2] concluded that HT had been used by 50% of women aged 50–64 and was used currently by around one-third. Use appeared to be influenced more strongly by a woman's medical or surgical history than by socioeconomic or lifestyle factors. For example, following bilateral oophorectomy the current usage was 66%, hysterectomy without removal of ovaries 48%, breast cancer 6%, diabetes 25%, heart disease 31% and stroke 24%. The average duration of use was 5.8 years. In fact, in one study, up to 30% of patients did not even collect their prescription from the pharmacy![1] A surprisingly large number of doctors fail to recommend HT to patients who might benefit from it[3]. Other factors associated with non-use of HT are concerns about side-effects, including bleeding, perceived risks such as breast cancer, and anxiety about weight gain. However, it is surely of note that when women are well informed about HT, the uptake is much greater[4] (Table 8.1). The common concerns about HT are discussed in the following sections.

Table 8.1   Prevalence of use of hormone replacement therapy by age group in menopausal and postmenopausal women doctors. Adapted from reference 4

	Current users		Ever-users		
	n	%	n	%	Total
All ages	344	37.8	472	51.9	909
Age groups (years)					
40–44	9	52.9	11	64.7	17
45–49	49	54.4	52	57.8	90
50–54	85	53.5	104	65.4	159
55–59	114	45.1	155	61.3	253
60–64	71	26.1	117	42.9	273
65–69	14	15.4	28	30.8	91
> 70	22	7.7	5	19.2	26

8.2   Many women discontinue treatment because of side-effects

Either estrogen or progestogen or both may cause side-effects (Table 8.2). Progestogenic side-effects only occur during the progestogen phase of treatment, while estrogenic side-effects can occur at any time in the cycle. In fact, many side-effects settle down after the first few weeks of treatment. If not, there are a number of strategies which may help (Table 8.3).

8.3   The older postmenopausal woman needs to be started on a low dose of estrogen to minimize side-effects

Estrogenic side-effects can be a particular problem for older women in need of HT who have been without estrogen for some

Table 8.2   Possible side-effects of estrogen and progestogen in HT

Side-effects of estrogen	Side-effects of progestogen
Fluid retention	PMS-type symptoms such as fluid retention, abdominal bloating, migraine, nausea, mood swings, irritability, tearfulness
Bloating	
Breast tenderness or enlargement	Breast tenderness
Nausea	Aching in the pelvis
Indigestion	Depression
Headaches	Acne
Leg cramps	Greasy skin/hair

PMS, premenstrual syndrome

years. They need to start on a very low 'priming' dose and gradually increase, over a few weeks, to therapeutic doses. This can be achieved by using patches cut into quarters, then halves and so on.

8.4   Altering the dose and delivery route can alleviate side-effects of progestogen

About 25% of women experience side-effects from progestogen. About 5% of these will find their symptoms sufficiently disabling to discontinue treatment. For these women, clinicians can experiment with the range of progestogens now available, in the expectation of finding an acceptable regimen (see Appendix).

The side-effects of progestogens may be worse with the androgenic progestogens, norethisterone and levonorgestrel. These are chemically derived from testosterone, and, with their greater similarity to the male sex hormone, may produce side-effects such as acne, greasy skin and hair, darkening of facial hair, and PMS-type symptoms such as bloating, headaches and depression.

Table 8.3   Current strategies available to minimize the side-effects of estrogen and progestogen

Estrogenic side-effects	Progestogenic side-effects
Persist with treatment for 12 weeks to allow side-effects to settle	Use the lowest dose of progestogen known to be effective for endometrial protection (Table 2.2)
Try gamolenic acid (Oil of Evening Primrose) for breast tenderness	Try taking half the oral dose morning and evening (cut tablet in half) to reduce the surge in blood levels seen with oral preparations
Take oral dose with food to minimize nausea and indigestion	
Lactose-free (non-oral route) preparations for women with lactose intolerance	Try a different type of progestogen. Changing from a testosterone to a progesterone derivative (MPA or dydrogesterone) may help women who experience androgenic side-effects
Reduce dose, but maintain bone-sparing dose	
In older women, prime with a low dose, gradually increase to therapeutic doses over a few weeks	Try a non-oral preparation, e.g. transdermal patch, vaginal gel or intrauterine device*
Change type of estrogen to estradiol or conjugated equine estrogens	Reduce the frequency of administration by using long-cycle therapy with progestogen for 14 days every 3 months
Change delivery route – oral, transdermal, nasal, vaginal or implant	In women 1 year postmenopausal, try continuous combined therapy which delivers a lower dose of progestogen
	Tibolone as an alternative to CCEPT

*In many countries, the Mirena intrauterine device, containing levonorgestrel, is only licensed for contraception and treating heavy periods. It produces an atrophic endometrium and can be used with oral or transdermal estrogen to provide CCEPT

The non-androgenic progestogens, dydrogesterone or MPA, may be a better option for some women.

8.5   No-bleed treatments increase long-term use of HT

For most women, one of the few benefits of reaching the menopause is the cessation of periods. It is understandable, therefore, that the idea of restarting bleeding (in the older postmenopausal woman), or prolonging it (perimenopausal women) is not popular. One study showed that nearly half of a group of previous HT users cited bleeding as a reason for discontinuing treatment[5].

The use of continuous/combined treatment (see Appendix), which produces an atrophic endometrium, is the way forward, and is the most suitable treatment for long-term use. This approach is suitable for:

- Women at least 1 year past the menopause

- Women using sequential treatment and who are over the age of 54 (the age at which, statistically, 80% will be at least 1 year postmenopause)

However, they must be advised of possible initial bleeding problems, reassured that most women achieve a period-free state with perseverance, and encouraged to consult about difficulties (see also Section 3.4).

8.6   The increased risk of breast cancer associated with HT use is lower than most women realize

Naturally women fear breast cancer, but many also believe that HT significantly increases the risk. In one survey, 40% of women thought they were most likely to die from breast cancer, and only 19% cited heart disease[6].

The reality is that about 8% will die from breast cancer and up to 60% from cardiovascular disease. Furthermore, 60% of women will suffer an osteoporotic fracture at some time, 17% being hip fractures which are associated with at least 25% mortality within 6 months in the elderly[7].

Numerous attempts have been made over the years to quantify the link between HT use and breast cancer. The results have shown various degrees of association and the picture has been confusing. However, in 1997, the Collaborative Group on Hormonal Factors in Breast Cancer produced an analysis of 51 scientific studies involving a total of over 160 000 women, some of whom had used or were using HT[8]. About one-third of these women had breast cancer. They concluded that, in women over 50, HT increased the risk of breast cancer by 2.3% for each year of use. However, the use of percentages or relative risk figures is difficult for most people to put into perspective. Much more understandable are absolute terms, and the results from this report translate to an extra two women developing breast cancer per 1000 after 5 years of use, and an extra six after 10 years.

However, larger more recent studies such as the Women's Health Initiative (WHI)[9] and the Million Women Study (MWS)[10] have further established the risk of HT and especially of combined estrogen and progestogen.

8.7 Risk of breast cancer may be greater with combined estrogen and progestogen

Before the WHI study there was strong evidence that HT was associated with an increased risk of breast cancer, but there were few data on the possible different effects of estrogen and progestogen and the various combinations or routes of administration. The combined estrogen and progestogen (CEPT) arm of the WHI study was stopped in June 2002 because of an unacceptable risk of breast cancer[9], (RR = 1.26 (0.83–1.92)) but the unopposed estrogen arm (conjugated equine estrogen (CEE)

0.625 mg daily) continues without apparently a significant increase in breast cancer risk. Further reports from WHI have indicated that CEPT was associated with the development of larger and more advanced tumors than in the placebo group[11], which is contrary to some previous reports.

The MWS is a large, observational study that examines the effects of specific types of HT on the incidence of, and mortality from, breast cancer in 828 923 postmenopausal women in the UK over a 5-year period. The National Health Service Breast Screening Programme, which invites all women in the UK aged 50–64 years for routine screening once every 3 years, was used to recruit the women. The average age of the women at recruitment was 55.9 years, with a mean period of follow-up of 2.6 years for analysis of the cancer incidence and 4.1 years for analyses of mortality. Overall, 50% of the women were ever-users of HT. The relative risk of breast cancer was significantly raised for current users of estrogen-only preparations (1.30 (1.21–1.40), $p < 0.0001$), estrogen/progestogen combinations (2.00 (1.88–2.12), $p < 0.0001$), and tibolone (1.45 (1.25–1.68), $p < 0.0001$). However, the magnitude of the relative risk of breast cancer varied significantly between these three HT types ($p < 0.0001$) and was substantially greater in users of CEPT than for other preparations. As with previous reports, the risk for current users was increased with total duration of HT, but was evident earlier than in previous reports at 1–2 years from starting treatment and past users were not at increased risk. The risk of dying from breast cancer was also increased (1.22 (1.00–1.48), $p = 0.05$).

Irrespective of the type of HT used, the risk of breast cancer decreased after cessation of use and returned to the same risk as for non-users by 5 years.

Because this study was so large, it was possible to analyze the effects of different types of HT. There was no difference in the risk of cancer with the type of estrogen (CEE or estradiol) or the route of administration – oral, transdermal or subcutaneous implant, or with type of progestogen – medroxyprogesterone acetate, norethisterone, norgestrel or levonorgestrel. There was no difference in risk between sequential and continuous combined regimens.

As with the WHI reports, much emphasis and publicity has been given to the relative risks and percentage increases of 30–200%, whereas absolute figures provide a more suitable perspective of the risk. The additional cancers associated with estrogen were only 1.5 after 5 years and 5 after 10 years and for CEPT the figures are 6 and 19, respectively, per 1000 women by the age of 65 years (Table 8.4; Figure 8.1). Or, put another way, a doctor would need to prescribe CEPT to 116 women for 5 years, or 53 women for 10 years, to see one extra case of breast cancer.

This is a very large study that has produced new and alarming data. Although it is an observational study, which epidemiologists

Table 8.4 Cumulative and excess incidence of invasive breast cancer in 1000 women who had never used and ever used HT, based on incidence rates typical of developed countries. Adapted with permission from reference 9

	Never users of HT	Duration of use of estrogen only (years)		Duration of use of estrogen–progestogen (years)	
		5	10	5	10
Up to age (years)					
50	18	18	18	18	18
55	27	28.5	29	34	34
60	38	39.5	43	44	57
65	50	51.5	55	56	69
Excessive cumulative incidence per 1000 HT users (95% CI)	0	1.5 (0–3)	5 (3–7)	6 (5–7)	19 (18–20)

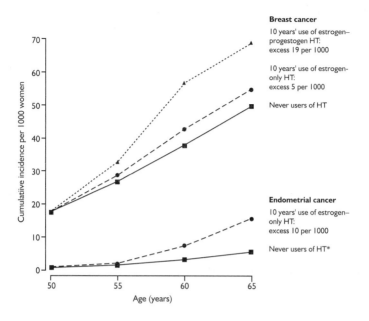

Figure 8.1

Estimated cumulative incidence of breast and endometrial cancer per 1000 women in developed countries who never used HT and who used HT for 10 years, beginning at age 50 years. *10 years' use of estrogen–progestogen HT estimated to result in little change in cumulative incidence of endometrial cancer. Reproduced from reference 9 with permission

usually consider to be unreliable due to confounding variables for which only a true, randomized, controlled trial can counter, it has the merit of very large numbers which probably does give it credibility. This study, together with reports from WHI and others[12] are now raising serious concerns about the merits of progestogen in CEPT. With an apparent four-fold greater risk of breast cancer compared with estrogen alone, the balance of this risk against the merit of protecting the endometrium (see Section 8.9), which is the only reason for giving progestogen, has now to be seriously considered. Indeed, in the discussion part of the MWS report it is suggested that there is little advantage to women with a uterus in using CEPT in preference to unopposed estrogen, since the risk of endometrial cancer from the latter is much less than the risk of breast cancer from combination therapy. This view would be absolutely counter to the perceived wisdom and teaching over the last 25 years and ignores the clinical implications other than just endometrial cancer. Unopposed estrogen will increase the risk of abnormal bleeding and pre-malignant endometrial pathology and will increase the risk for gynecological consultation, endometrial investigations and hysterectomy. At a time when hysterectomy rates may be declining, it would be ironic if this trend reverses so that women may more safely have unopposed estrogen therapy.

8.8 Tibolone seems to have a similar, though less potent, effect on breast cancer risk compared with combined estrogen and progestogen therapy (CEPT)

Another surprising finding from MWS was an increased risk of breast cancer associated with tibolone (RR = 1.45 (1.25–1.68), $p < 0.0001$) but this was less than with CEPT. This synthetic hormone which has been available for 25 years has a mixture of estrogenic, progestogenic and androgenic actions and data, up until this report, had suggested that it should cause less breast stimulation than conventional HT. It certainly causes minimal change in mammographic breast density, in contrast to CEPT regimens[13], which may allow earlier detection of breast cancer (Figure 8.2). The effect of tibolone on breast cancer will be better tested in a 5-year randomized, placebo-controlled trial in women who have previously had invasive breast cancer. The trial (LIBERATE) is currently at the enrolment phase.

8.9 Breast cancer risk related to body weight

The increased risk of breast cancer with larger exposure to HT seems to be limited in most studies to women of normal or low

Before   **6 months HT**

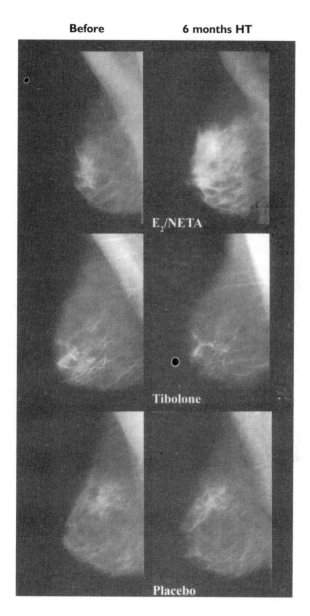

Figure 8.2

Changes in mammographic density in three individual women according to treatment. Mammograms were obtained before *(left)* and after *(right)* 6 months of therapy. The woman receiving estradiol/norethisterone acetate (E$_2$/NETA) had an apparent increase in breast density, whereas no change was recorded in the women on tibolone and placebo treatment. Reproduced with permission from reference 13

BMI (< 25 kg/m²). Conversely, being overweight is an independent risk factor for breast cancer due to the extra production of estrogen in adipose tissue.

Other risk factors for breast cancer (Table 8.5) help to put the effects of HT into perspective.

The MWS and another recent study[12] have refuted previous suggestions that breast cancers occurring during HT are less advanced and have a better prognosis.

Table 8.5   Established and possible risk factors for breast cancer. Adapted with permission from McPherson K, Steel CM, Dixon JM. Breast cancer – epidemiology, risk factors and genetics. *Br Med J* 2000;321:624–8

Factor	Relative risk	High-risk group
Age	> 10	elderly
Geographical location	5	developed country
Age at menarche	3	menarche before 11
Age at menopause	1.14	menopause after 55
Age at first full pregnancy	1.48	pregnancy after 30
Family history	≥ 2	breast cancer in first-degree relative when young
Previous benign disease	4–5	atypical hyperplasia
Cancer in other breast	> 4	
Socioeconomic group	2	groups I and II
Diet	1.5	high intake of saturated fat
Body weight		
premenopausal	0.7	body mass index > 35
postmenopausal	1.48	body mass index > 30
Alcohol consumption	1.16	2 units per day
Exposure to ionizing radiation	3	abnormal exposure in young females after age 10
Oral contraceptive	1.24	current and recent use
Hormone therapy	1.26–2.0	current use postmenopause

These figures put into perspective the increased breast and endometrial cancer risk associated with HT use and, for each individual woman, this needs to be balanced against the potential benefits of HT in reducing osteoporosis and possibly of cardiovascular disease and Alzheimer's disease.

The perimenopausal woman may need to use HT for about 5 years for relief of menopausal symptoms, but, if there are no particular risk factors for osteoporosis or heart disease, a break from HT may then be appropriate. This would minimize any breast cancer risk, and she can then consider restarting at say age 60, by which time her increased breast cancer risk will have fallen to non-user levels, and she can benefit from the long-term protection afforded by HT. For further discussion of such strategies see Section 5.11.

8.10   Other factors and lifestyle present greater risk of breast cancer than HT

HT is a relatively low-risk factor for breast cancer compared to several other common situations, but far less publicity is given to the effect of alcohol or having a first baby over the age of 30 years, for example (Table 8.5).

8.11   Breast cancer patients can be treated with alternatives to HT

Women who have been diagnosed with breast cancer are not generally prescribed HT, given the *possible* growth-promoting effects of estrogen on any dormant malignant cells. However, the situation is not at all clear, and many oncologists are now allowing such women to try HT, without as yet any reported evidence of harm. Indeed, there are some reports of a lower risk of further disease, and this possibility is currently under investigation.

The effect of chemotherapy on the ovaries may induce a premature menopause and acute menopausal symptoms. In addition, tamoxifen, which is usually given to women with estrogen receptor-positive breast cancer, has an antiestrogenic effect not only on breast, but also in the brain, causing distressing hot flushes. Tamoxifen is a selective estrogen receptor modulator (SERM – see Section 2.7) and in some aspects is an effective form of HT, with prevention of osteoporosis in particular. Raloxifene (Evista®), a more recent SERM is licensed for the prevention and treatment of osteoporosis and, like tamoxifen, positively alters the blood lipid profile, although whether this translates into a decrease in cardiovascular disease has yet to be established. There are, however, encouraging data showing a significant reduction in the incidence of breast cancer in raloxifene users compared to controls[14]. Bisphosphonates are another option for the treatment or prevention of osteoporosis (Section 5.6).

Given the availability of these long-term alternatives to estrogen treatment, the management of acute menopausal symptoms, and especially the hot flushes associated with tamoxifen, becomes the main problem. Non-systemic vaginal estrogen preparations can treat urogenital symptoms, and progestogens (norethisterone 5 mg or megestrol acetate 60 mg daily) have been shown to alleviate hot flushes and sweats[15,16]. (See Section 4.4 for further comments about non-estrogen treatment of flushes.) Avoiding triggers such as overheating, alcohol, spicy foods, tea and coffee is advisable. Some women find natural therapies and dietary approaches to be helpful (see Chapter 9).

For some women, the above strategies will not be effective or satisfactory, so that the use of HT becomes a consideration.

8.12 Using progestogens along with estrogens has largely eliminated the risk of endometrial cancer from HT use

This topic was covered in Section 2.4, and can be summarized as follows:

- Unopposed estrogen increases the risk of endometrial hyperplasia and hence endometrial cancer

- This increased risk lasts for several years after treatment is stopped

- Giving a progestogen at a suitable dose for 10–14 days each month reduces the risk of hyperplasia

- Sequential treatment can be used for 5 years after the menopause without increased risk of endometrial cancer

- Continuous/combined therapy keeps the endometrium thin and atrophic and, with long-term use, may even reduce the risk of endometrial cancer compared to non-users

- Women who are taking sequential HT, and are more than 1 year past the menopause, should be advised of the better protective effect of continuous combined HT and invited to switch[17]

8.13　The bleeding problem in women taking HT

This topic was also covered in Sections 3.4 and 8.5.

- Women need to be advised before starting that unsatisfactory or abnormal bleeding is a common problem during HT, particularly during the first few months

- Sequential regimens should provide a regular and predictable bleed

- About 5% of women will not have a bleed during sequential therapy. This does not matter and indicates that the endometrium has lost the ability to respond. Such women do not need to be investigated, but should continue to take the progestogen as well as the estrogen

- During both sequential and continuous combined therapy abnormal bleeding is usually due to persistent ovarian activity, which often can be overcome by altering the dose of estrogen and/or progestogen

- Continued abnormal bleeding requires investigation to exclude endometrial pathology

- Developments of the intrauterine progestogen-releasing device will provide better control of the endometrium

- The SERM raloxifene does not stimulate the endometrium and is suitable for older postmenopausal women for osteoporosis prevention

8.14 Contrary to popular belief, HT does not cause weight gain

Many women think that using HT will increase their weight, and cite this as a reason for not taking it. However, a Cochrane analysis[18] of 22 separate randomized controlled studies has shown that there is no difference in weight gain between women on HT and those not on it. For example, in the well-designed PEPI investigation, nearly 900 women were randomly assigned to a placebo or various regimens of HT. After 3 years, those who took HT were, on average, 1 kg lighter than those on the placebo[19].

Logically, if estrogen were to cause an increase in weight, then menopausal women should lose weight as their estrogen levels decline. In fact, the opposite happens. Women tend both to put on weight and to find it more difficult to lose it, for two reasons. First, in middle age, the metabolic rate goes down. The energy intake recommended for women over 50 is 1900 kcal, compared with 2200 kcal in younger women. If a 50+ woman continues to eat this extra 300 kcal per day, she can put on about 30 lbs in weight in a year! Second, older women are often less active than before, so consuming fewer calories. Women also change shape, with fat being moved from their breasts and buttocks to the abdomen. This is 'middle-age spread', and HT reverses it to some extent.

In summary, it is not HT, which is responsible for weight gain, but the natural bodily changes occurring at this age. Reduced food consumption and exercise are the only ways to keep weight down.

However, a small minority of women experience significant gains in weight after starting HT and find it difficult to lose it after stopping. The reasons for this are not clear. Fluid retention has been discounted and one theory is that estrogen stimulates the appetite in such women.

8.15 There is a small increase in risk of deep vein thrombosis with HT

A deep vein thrombosis (DVT) occurs when a blood clot forms in a vein, usually in the leg, blocking the flow of blood back from the leg and causing swelling and tenderness. If some of the clot breaks off, it may travel to the heart and thence to the lung causing a pulmonary embolus, which can be fatal. However, DVT is a rare condition affecting only about one woman per 10 000 per year.

HT can alter hepatic production of coagulation and fibrinolytic factors, which increase the risk of thrombosis by a factor of about 3[20]. This translates to an extra two affected women per 10 000 per year, or one per 5000 per year. The increased risk is greatest during the first year of treatment, and death resulting from DVT leading to pulmonary embolism is rare. In women with no risk factors for DVT, this tiny increase has to be set against the dangers of osteoporosis. A non-oral route carries less risk as it bypasses the liver and avoids the negative effects on clotting mechanisms seen with oral treatment (Section 6.7, Table 6.2). A recent report comparing the incidence of venous thrombosis (VTE) in users of oral and transdermal HT preparations in France found that only those using oral HT were at increased risk[21]. The estimated risk for VTE in current users of oral HT compared with transdermal was 4.0 (1.9–8.3). Obesity and smoking add to the risk of DVT and it is estimated that about 6% of the general population carry inherited risk factors. Women with a previous or family history of the condition should have a thrombophilia screen before starting HT to establish if they are naturally at increased risk. However, there are no data on the use of HT in women who are shown to have an inherited disposition to DVT, but one study of women with a previously verified DVT or pulmonary embolism who were given estradiol 2 mg and norethisterone 1 mg daily or a placebo, was stopped early because of accumulating evidence about the risk of DVT with HT[22].

8.16 Most of the contraindications in the data sheets which accompany HT have been extrapolated from those for the contraceptive pill – there are actually very few absolute contraindications to its use

In 1997, Hartmann and Huber[23] summarized the numerous contraindications to HT use listed in the data sheets of five currently available estrogen replacement preparations. These included cardiovascular disease, diabetes, endometriosis, liver diseases and hormone-dependent tumors. They indicated that these had been lifted from the data sheets of oral contraceptives, and extrapolated to HT, thus erroneously influencing the prescribing decisions of doctors, and frightening women who read the information contained in the drug packet. In fact, diabetes and possibly cardiovascular disease could be indications for HT, although the latter is now rather controversial.

The synthetic estrogen used in the contraceptive pill, ethinylestradiol, is much more potent than the natural estrogens used in HT and is up to 200 times more effective in inhibiting production of the pituitary follicle stimulating hormone necessary for ovulation. This, of course, is why it is such an effective contraceptive. The thrombogenic effect on the liver is also more marked. The estrogens used in HT have quite different pharmacological characteristics and, in fact, there are very few contraindications to HT use (Tables 8.6–8.8).

Table 8.6   Specific medical conditions and HT

Hypertension	generally no change with HT and small decreases in blood pressure have been reported[24]. Any rise in blood pressure is more likely to be caused by weight gain rather than HT. Well-controlled hypertension is not a contraindication. (Rarely, oral HT may provoke an increase in blood pressure, but if so, it occurs within the first 2–3 months)
Ovarian cancer	limited data suggesting long-term use of unopposed estrogen may slightly increase risk of developing ovarian cancer. No increase in risk of recurrence except possibly for the rare endometrioid ovarian cancer
Cervical cancer	there is no increased risk of cervical cancer, nor is there any evidence that progression from premalignant to malignant disease is hastened. A history of abnormal smears or of cervical cancer is not a contraindication
Endometriosis*	there is a risk that HT might stimulate endometrial deposits left after a pelvic clearance. CCEPT or tibolone are recommended to avoid this, and the lowest dose of estrogen required to combat symptoms should be used. Any symptoms indicating recurrence should be investigated
Endometrial hyperplasia*	this should be monitored and HT should contain adequate progestogen, given for at least 12 days every 4-week cycle or continuously. Persistent hyperplasia or atypical features require gynecologist advice
Fibroids	theoretically, HT could stimulate growth of fibroids but this does not seem to be a major problem
Diabetes*	estradiol decreases insulin levels and insulin resistance. Diabetic women may benefit from HT and their control may need to be reassessed

continued

149

Gall bladder disease*	HT is not contraindicated but a non-oral route should be used to avoid the liver. Oral therapy may unmask existing undiagnosed disease
Varicose veins	HT is not contraindicated unless the woman is undergoing surgery, which doubles the risk of DVT, when either HT should be stopped several weeks before surgery or prophylactic anticoagulation given before and for several days after the operation
Epilepsy*	some anti-epileptic drugs induce liver enzymes. A non-oral route for HT would reduce the possibility of interference with blood levels of the anti-epileptic medication
Raised blood triglycerides	a non-oral route is preferable as some oral estrogens elevate triglycerides
Melanoma	malignant melanoma is increasing, but there is no clinical evidence that HT affects the disease or provokes malignant progression of benign moles
Systemic lupus erythematosis (SLE)*	often treated with long-term steroids with increased risk of osteoporosis for which HT would be helpful. Traditional fear that HT will cause flare up, but evidence is scarce. Previous VTE or positive for lupus anticoagulant would be contraindication for HT
Otosclerosis	occasional reports of worsening during pregnancy and with oral contraception but no evidence of detrimental effect with HT
Migraine	often triggered by fluctuating hormone levels during menstrual cycle. May be provoked by progestogen phase of CSEPT. Transdermal administration produces more stable circulating levels and may be less likely to provoke or exacerbate migraine. Continuous combined regimens reduce fluctuations and the intrauterine levonorgestrel-releasing device may be a good option
Thyroid disease	HT not contraindicated but dose of thyroxine may need adjustment as thyroxine binding globulin levels increased by estrogen
Asthma	no evidence that HT affects asthma
Liver disease*	a non-oral route is advisable to avoid the first-pass effects. Limited data on effect of HT

DVT, deep vein thrombosis; VTE, venous thromboembolism; *special considerations apply

Table 8.7   Absolute contraindications to HT

Severe acute liver disease

Endometrial or breast cancer with recurrence

Active venous thromboembolism

Table 8.8   Relative contraindications to HT

Abnormal vaginal bleeding

Uninvestigated breast lump

Previous endometrial or breast cancer

Strong family history of breast cancer

Previous venous thromboembolism

Family history of thromboembolism

Proven coronary heart disease

References

1.   Hammond CB. Women's concerns with hormone replacement therapy – compliance issues. *Fertil Steril* 1994;62(Suppl 2):157s–60s

2.   Million Women Study Collaborators. Patterns of use of hormone replacement therapy in one million women in Britain, 1996–2002. *Br J Obstet Gynaecol* 2002;109:1319–30

3.   Newton KM, LaCroix AZ, Leveille SG, *et al*. The physician's role in women's decision making about hormone replacement therapy. *Obstet Gynaecol* 1998;92:580–4

4. Isaacs AJ, Britton AR, McPherson K. Utilisation of hormone replacement therapy by women doctors. *Br Med J* 1995;311:1399–401

5. Karakoc B, Erenus M. Compliance considerations with hormone replacement therapy. *Menopause* 1998;5:102–6

6. Purdie DW. Potential applications of SERMS. In *SERMS, a New Choice for Postmenopausal Health. Proceedings of a Satellite Symposium at the 6th Bath Conference on Osteoporosis.* 1998:10–12

7. Cummings SR, Black DM, Rubin SM. Lifetime risks of hip and Colles' fractures and coronary heart disease in postmenopausal women. *Arch Intern Med* 1989;149:2445–8

8. The Collaborative Group on Hormonal Factors in Breast Cancer. Hormone replacement therapy and breast cancer. *Lancet* 1997;350:1047–5

9. Writing Group for the Women's Health Initiative Investigators. Risks and benefits of estrogen plus progestin in healthy post-menopausal women: principal results from the Women's Health Initiative randomized controlled trial. *J Am Med Assoc* 2002;288:321–33

10. Million Women Study Collaborators. Breast cancer and hormone-replacement therapy in the Million Women Study. *Lancet* 2003;362:419–27

11. Chlebowski RT, Hendrix SL, Langer RD, *et al.* for the WHI Investigators. Influence of estrogen plus progestin on breast cancer and mammography in healthy postmenopausal women: the Women's Health Initiative randomized controlled trial. *J Am Med Assoc* 2003;289:3243–53

12. Li CI, Malone KE, Porter PL, *et al*. Relationship between long durations and different regimens of hormone therapy and risk of breast cancer. *J Am Med Assoc* 2003;289:3254–63

13. Lundstrom E, Christow A, Kersemaekers, *et al*. Effects of tibolone and continuous combined hormone replacement therapy on mammographic dsnsity. *Am J Obstet Gynecol* 2002;186;717–22

14. Cummings SR, Eckert S, Krueger KA, *et al*. The effect of raloxifene on risk of breast cancer in postmenopausal women: results from the MORE randomized trial. Multiple Outcomes in Raloxifene Evaluation. *J Am Med Assoc* 1999;281:2189–97

15. Paterson MEL. A randomised double blind cross over trial into the effect of norethisterone on climacteric symptoms and biochemical profiles. *Br J Obstet Gynaecol* 1992;89:464–72

16. Farish E, Barnes JF, O'Donoghue F, *et al*. The role of megestrol acetate as an alternative to conventional hormone replacement therapy. *Climacteric* 2000;3:125–34

17. Wells M, Sturdee DW, Barlow DH, *et al*. The endometrial response to long term continuous combined oestrogen-progestogen replacement therapy: a follow-up study. *Br Med J* 2002;325:239–42

18. Norman RJ, Flight IHK, Rees MCP. Oestrogen and progestogen hormone replacement therapy for peri-menopausal and post-menopausal women: weight and body fat distribution (Cochrane Review). *The Cochrane Library*, Issue 3, 2001. Update software Ltd.

19. Working Group for the PEPI Trial. Effects of estrogen or estrogen/progestin regimens on heart disease risk factors in post-

menopausal women: the Postmenopausal Estrogen/Progestin Intervention (PEPI) Trial. *J Am Med Assoc* 1995;273:199–208

20. Daly E, Vessey MP, Hawkins MM, *et al*. Risk of venous thrombo-embolism in users of hormone replacement therapy. *Lancet* 1996;348:977–80

21. Scarabin P-Y, Oger E, Plu-Bureau G; on behalf of the EStrogen and THromboEmbolism Risk (ESTHER) Study Group. Differential association of oral and transdermal oestrogen-replacement therapy with venous thromboembolism risk. *Lancet* 2003;362:428–32

22. Hoibraaten E, Qvigstad E, Andersen TO, *et al*. The effects of hormone replacement therapy (HRT) on haemostatic variables in women with previous venous thromboembolism – results from a randomized double-blind, clinical trial. *Thromb Haemostat* 2001;85:775–81

23. Hartmann BW, Huber C. The mythology of hormone replace-ment therapy. *Br J Obstet Gynaecol* 1997;104:163–8

24. Lip GY, Beevers M, Churchill D, Beevers DG. Hormone replacement therapy and blood pressure in hypertensive women. *J Hum Hypertens* 1994;8:491–4

Chapter 9

Current attitudes to HT

9.1 Adverse media reporting has fuelled scepticism about HT

Few women use HT. Numerous surveys have shown that, among those who try it, the discontinuation rate is high, varying between 20 and 60%, depending on the country and study. There are several reasons for this – they do not feel better, concerns about safety and side-effects, fear of cancer, the feeling that it is not natural, a belief that it will cause weight gain, and the continuation or re-establishment of bleeding. In addition, the long-term benefits of HT are now less certain.

For women, important sources of information about HT are the media and their general practitioner. The media, mindful of the fact that bad news sells, tend to concentrate on 'scare' stories, and to capitalize on their readers' lack of knowledge of the full medical context of the data being presented. Thus, readers are given an unbalanced viewpoint which plays on their fears. Two examples of media representation are:

- Banner headlines (such as those in Figure 9.1) which presented data from the WHI study as increased relative risk of heart disease of 29%, breast cancer 26% and stroke 41%, suggesting a much greater increase than the absolute figures of 7, 8 and 18 extra cases, respectively, per 10 000 women per year. Relative risk is a difficult concept to understand and requires knowledge of the underlying risk of the condition for the figures to be put into a clearer perspective

- A press report whose author wrongly quoted the risk of breast cancer on HT as being 1000 times greater than it actually is. Forced by vigorous protestations from medical experts to take back her statement, she published a retraction in a small corner of an inside page of the newspaper. The damage had already been done

It is not always easy, therefore, for women to obtain appropriate balanced advice or reassurance about HT and its effects, and

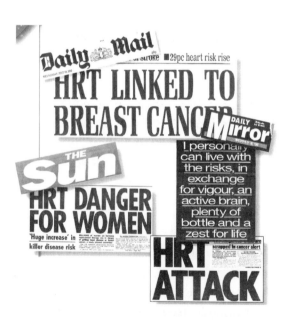

Figure 9.1

Examples of newspaper headlines following the reports from the Women's Health Initiative Study

Table 9.1 Reasons for telephone help-line enquiries from current users of hormone replacement therapy (V. Godfree, M. I. Whitehead, personal communication)

Reason	%
HT not controlling the symptoms	20
Bleeding problems	15
PMS-type side-effects of HT	10
Weight gain	10
Safety concerns	10
Information on period-free HT	10
Duration of HT	7
Headaches	4
Breast tenderness	3
Other side-effects	2

PMS, premenstrual syndrome

unrelieved concerns are a common cause for stopping treatment. Telephone help-lines can be particularly helpful (Table 9.1).

9.2 General practitioners are often confused by the information from the drug companies

Accurate information about HT is an important factor in patient acceptance, with lack of knowledge being more likely to lead to rejection of treatment and non-compliance[1].

Women doctors might be expected to have a greater comprehension of the risk/benefit ratio for HT, and indeed this is well illustrated by the fact that uptake and continuation of HT is relatively high among female general practitioners, who presumably are well-informed[2] (see Table 8.1). Similarly, a Swedish study reported even higher rates of use among postmenopausal female gynecologists and general practitioners of 88% and 72%, respectively[3].

The interest and support of health professionals has been shown to be significant in improving compliance. Some general practices have succeeded in raising their long-term compliance rates to over 85%[4,5], but, in general, prescribing practices are very patchy. General practitioners are more likely to prescribe for perimenopausal and recently menopausal women, but are reluctant to advocate long-term use.

While nearly all the general practitioners and gynecologists in one survey knew that HT protected against osteoporosis[6], a much smaller percentage (only 7% in the case of general practitioners) would prescribe it for over 10 years. The use of HT for osteoporosis is not well established, and even when women are found to be at increased risk of osteoporosis and fracture, a large proportion will still reject the opportunity of taking HT or will stop after a short time[7,8]. A survey in the UK[6] showed that HT was not routinely offered to women with a history of fracture or vascular problems by their general practitioner, and that women with heart disease, diabetes and high blood pressure were less likely to receive it, unless they had a hysterectomy. This surgical intervention appeared to alert general practitioners to the advisability of HT.

General practitioners are not always clear about the benefits and risks of HT and this uncertainty is conveyed to their patients. One probable reason for this stems from the pharmaceutical data sheets of HT regimens produced by the manufacturers[9]. As already mentioned (Section 8.13), the contraindications to HT were taken uncritically from the data sheets of oral contraceptives, which led to the erroneous belief that HT should not be prescribed for, among other conditions, hypertension and high fat levels in the blood. Similarly, systematic review of the medical literature shows that diabetes, chronic liver disease, endometriosis, some cases of treated cancer of the endometrium and breast, melanoma and otosclerosis are not contraindications to HT. The authors of the study state:

'The information in the pharmaceutical data sheets of HT regimens should be modified as more accurate information could influence how these preparations are prescribed by doctors as well as affect patient compliance.'

The demographic changes described in Chapter 1 highlight the urgency of the problem. At the start of a new millennium, women can expect to live on average for 33 years after the menopause in a state of relative estrogen deficiency. Many of these women will develop osteoporosis, Alzheimer's disease and colon cancer, in addition to a reduced quality of life due to the symptoms and effects of estrogen deficiency. The personal and public costs are huge. The ability of HT to ameliorate these conditions, means that it can be much more than a short-term solution to acute menopausal distress. Needless to say, physicians must themselves be cognisant of the progress being made in this field. It is incumbent on doctors and other health professionals to inform their patients of the benefits, especially in the long term, of HT, and to alert them to potential risks and side-effects, to listen to their concerns and, if they choose to try HT, to support them in finding a suitable regimen. HT can be part of a comprehensive program of disease prevention for women in their later years, alongside mammography, cardiovascular assessment and bone density measurement.

9.3 Possible alternatives to HT, especially plant estrogens, are the subject of considerable publicity, but little research

Phytoestrogens

The reluctance on the part of many women to use HT has led to an interest in alternative treatments for menopausal symptoms. Around 40% of women in the Western world are taking dietary supplements in the form of herbal and vitamin tablets and this is now a multimillion dollar industry. The substances which have received most attention are the *phytoestrogens*. The name phytoestrogen just means plant (phyto) estrogen, i.e. chemicals found in plants, which exert weak estrogenic effects. There are two main types, the lignans, found in linseeds, whole grains, fruits and vegetables, and the *isoflavones*, found in soy beans and other leguminous seeds. The isoflavones have been more extensively investigated than the lignans, especially genistein, daidzein and equol, the phytoestrogens found in large quantities in soy products.

Epidemiological studies reveal that the chronic diseases of Western postmenopausal women, such as breast and colon cancer, heart disease and osteoporosis, are less prevalent in Pacific Rim countries, especially Japan, where soy foods form a major part of the diet. In addition, Japanese women are often reported to suffer less from acute menopausal symptoms and there is not even a word in Japanese for flush! In reality they do experience hot flushes[10], although it may be that there are cultural taboos against reporting them. However, this has stimulated a flurry of interest, both in the lay and scientific communities, in the possible protective role of these plant compounds.

Research using animals has indicated that phytoestrogens may have a beneficial effect against cardiovascular disease and osteoporosis. For example, addition of soy to the diet of monkeys was shown to have cardioprotective effects (reduction of total plasma cholesterol and atherosclerotic deposits, and relaxation of coronary arteries)[11]. Studies in rats from whom the ovaries have been removed, have indicated that daidzein has similar effects to estrogen replacement therapy in preserving bone mineral density[12].

However, research into the application of such observations to humans is in its infancy, and findings to date have been conflicting. Studies have used different amounts of phyto-estrogens from different sources, have administered them for different lengths of time and have used different background diets.

This makes comparisons difficult and could explain the diversity of results.

Several studies have indicated that a dietary intake of about 25 g per day of soy protein (considerably more than in the average Western diet), along with a low-fat diet results in clinically significant reductions in blood cholesterol[13]. This has been countered by other studies which show that supplementing the diet with tablets containing phytoestrogens did not affect cholesterol levels[14,15].

With regard to osteoporosis, the data are scant. One study found an increase of 5% in bone mineral content in women treated with soy[16], and a synthetic isoflavone derivative, ipriflavone, appears to preserve bone mass and may increase the effect of estrogen on bones[17]. It is available in some countries for the management of osteoporosis, and is the subject of an ongoing multicenter, European trial for its effect on the risk of vertebral fracture in postmenopausal women.

There is some evidence that phytoestrogens alleviate hot flushes to a limited extent. A reduction of 45% has been reported with soy, compared with 70% and 30%, respectively, with estrogen and placebo[16,18,19] (Figure 9.2). However, one study of 155 breast cancer survivors who suffered from severe flushing found that the soy product was no more effective than the placebo[20]. In studies such as these, the placebo effect is marked[21]. This means that symptoms improve when an inert substance is given, as long as the patient believes they are being treated. It is an unexplained phenomenon in all therapies, and is one for which careful controls have to be in-built when designing a research study. The placebo effect lasts for about 3 months after which improvement stops and the symptoms return. A recent review of the use of phytoe-strogens at the menopause[22] concluded that, 'There is no evidence that it's better than placebo'.

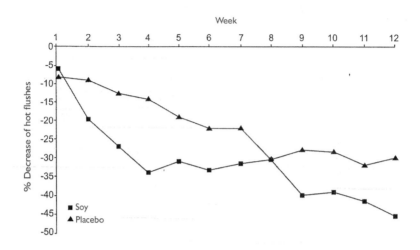

Figure 9.2

Weekly decrease (%) in the number of hot flushes experienced by women taking either soy protein or a placebo. The difference was significant after week 2, with the exception of week 8. Reproduced from reference 19 with permission

There is also considerable interest in the possible protective effects of phytoestrogens against cancer, especially breast cancer, again stimulated by the observed low cancer rates in populations with a phytoestrogen-rich diet. Table 9.2 summarizes some of the possible mechanisms of action of phytoestrogens on tissues, but it must be emphasized that these results are derived from animal or test-tube studies and that no conclusive clinical trials on humans have been carried out. It is not therefore possible to extrapolate these findings to humans, although much evidence suggests that further investigation could be fruitful.

In the meantime, however, no harm will come to women who increase their intake of phytoestrogens by eating more of the foods in which they are abundant. Quite the opposite, these foods are recommended by nutritionists as being an important part of a healthy diet, and if women also find that they provide some relief from menopausal symptoms, so much the better.

Table 9.2   Summary of the possible biochemical effects of phytoestrogens and the therapeutic implications

Biochemical effect	Possible therapeutic consequences
Estrogenic and antiestrogenic effects	like SERMs (Section 2.7), may inhibit effects of estrogen in the breast and uterus, while providing cardiovascular and skeletal protection
Action on pituitary hormones resulting in an increase in length of the menstrual cycle	may, over a lifetime, reduce the exposure to estrogen of breast tissues and hence reduce cancer risk. Could explain the lower rates of breast cancer in Asian populations
Inhibition of enzymes involved in estrogen synthesis	as above
Stimulation of synthesis of plasma estrogen-binding proteins by the liver	less estrogen is 'free' in the blood to exert its effects, hence reducing estrogen exposure as above
Inhibition of the activity of enzymes involved in cell division and proliferation	may inhibit the growth of cancer cells
Inhibition of the growth of new blood vessels (angiogenesis)	cancers need to develop their own blood vessels in order to increase in size
Antioxidant activity	counteracts the effects of free radicals, i.e. highly reactive compounds which can cause carcinogenic changes in DNA
Inhibition of the early stages of tumor development	reduction in carcinogenesis

Other proposed remedies

Other alternative menopausal remedies for which claims have been made are black cohosh, agnus castus, Siberian ginseng, dong quai, evening primrose oil, wild yam and St. John's Wort. The only one which has been scientifically studied is black cohosh (*Cimicifuga racemosa*), but a review of four randomized controlled trials concluded that, despite plausible mechanisms of action, there was no compelling evidence for an effect on menopausal symptoms[23]. Short-term side-effects include gastrointestinal upsets and rashes[24], but long-term side-effects are unknown, so it is recommended that it be used for only 6 months. Further rigorous clinical trials are urgently needed.

Evening primrose oil has been shown to be effective for breast tenderness but of no value in alleviating menopausal symptoms[25]. Women with contraindications to estrogen should avoid ginseng as it has estrogenic effects.

Progesterone cream (Progest®) has been heavily promoted both in the UK and the USA[26] and is the subject of some debate and controversy. A randomized controlled trial, involving over 100 women, found an improvement in 83% of those in the treatment group who had experienced hot flushes, compared with 19% of the placebo group[27]. However, no effect on bone mineral density was found. This well-designed study contradicts the assertions that progesterone cream has a protective effect on bone[26]. Other studies found that insufficient progesterone is absorbed to attain the blood levels required to protect the endometrium or have any significant clinical effect[28,29].

None of the products or preparations mentioned in this Section have a license for the treatment of postmenopausal women, but they remain very popular and women are spending a large amount of money on them. However, there is no regulation or quality control of many of the herbal products and little information on their possible mode of action or potential side-effects. In contrast, all the licensed HT preparations have had to undergo very extensive and scientifically valid research in order to pass the close scrutiny of the medical licensing authorities, so that one can be confident that the claims of benefit are well proven. Until the manufacturers of these non-medical supplements provide similar evidence, it is not appropriate to be recommending their use.

9.4 Future developments in HT may increase patient acceptability and continuance

Many questions remain to be answered about HT. Further results of the ongoing international, prospective trials into the effects on cardiovascular disease (Chapter 6) will be reported over the next few years. The outcome of the unopposed estrogen arm of the WHI will be especially interesting if this shows significantly different effects to those found in the combined estrogen and progestogen group. More research is needed to elucidate the findings of both the WHI and HERS studies (Section 6.9) which indicated an adverse effect in women, with or without established cardiovascular disease. Unfortunately, the MRC WISDOM study has been stopped[30].

The exciting early results regarding the possible reduction of risk of Alzheimer's disease have not been confirmed by WHI, and in women over the age of 75 years there may be an increased risk with HT[31], but these findings need further research.

The risk of breast cancer with CEPT especially is greater than previously thought following the further analyses from the WHI study and the recent Million Women Study. It is likely that there will therefore be less support for long-term HT usage and advice to limit duration for symptom relief. However, there are good data showing that estrogen increases bone mineral density, and recent evidence that it actually reduces hip fracture risk as well as other fractures. Since fracture risk is proportional to bone density it would seem self-evident, but it has only now been convincingly clinically demonstrated.

The research into designer hormones (SERMs) will continue and the results of the RUTH trial into raloxifene and the heart (Section 6.12) are awaited.

New formulations of HT containing new progestogens and smaller, improved patches will become available. It seems doubtful if any further routes of administration can be identified!

Individualization of treatment, based on medical history and current needs will become the watchword, with age being no barrier to successful treatment. The idea that HT can be used at different stages of a woman's postmenopausal life, that she can start it in the perimenopausal years, stop and then continue later at a lower dose, using no-bleed regimens, may gain wider acceptability. HT probably does not significantly increase life span, but it can certainly improve well-being and 'add life to the years'.

9.5   Final thoughts

- Although the human female is unique in the animal kingdom in having a menopause, it is still a natural life event

- Loss of ovarian production of estrogen is the basic cause of the various symptoms and physical effects attributed to the menopause

- There is a wide spectrum of individual responses to the menopause

- HT is most suitable for those with:
  - menopausal symptoms that are affecting the quality of life
  - increased risk of osteoporosis

- Long-term benefits of HT require long-term use

- There is no single preparation that is suitable for all women

- The lowest effective dose should be prescribed, re-evaluated annually and adjusted to the woman's needs and clinical response

- Low-dose continuous combined HT regimens are most likely to be acceptable for the long term

- Women need to be well informed and updated about the risks and benefits of HT and the merits of continuing therapy should be regularly evaluated

- New data on the risks and benefits of HT need to be put into appropriate perspective. Absolute or excess risk is usually easier to understand than percentage increase or relative risk

- Women who are taking HT need to have easy access to, and confidence in, their medical support

- Not every woman needs or will necessarily benefit from HT

- HT is not a panacea for all the problems of middle and later life

- To date, there is no evidence that unlicensed dietary supplements have any beneficial effects that are comparable to HT

- A healthy lifestyle is more important for most women

A final thought from a pioneer for improving the quality of life of older women:

'A woman in the autumn of her years deserves an Indian summer rather than a winter of discontent'

Robert Greenblatt

References

1. Jensen LB, Hilden J. Sociological and behavioural characteristics of perimenopausal women with an express attitude to hormone substitution therapy. *Maturitas* 1996;23:73–83

2. Isaacs AJ, Britton AR, McPherson K. Utilisation of hormone replacement therapy by women doctors. *Br Med J* 1995;311:1399–401

3. Andersson K, Pedersen AT, Mattson LA, Milson I. Swedish gynaecologists' and general practitioners' views on the climacteric period: knowledge, attitudes and management strategies. *Acta Obstet Gynaecol Scand* 1998;77:909–16

4. Coope J, Marsh J. Can we improve compliance with long-term HT? *Maturitas* 1992;15:151–8

5. Halbert DR, Lloyd T, Rollings N, *et al.* Hormone replacement therapy usage: a 10-year experience of a solo practitioner. *Maturitas* 1998;29:67–73

6. Norman SG, Studd JWW. A survey of views on hormone replacement therapy. *Br J Obstet Gynaecol* 1994;101:879–87

7. Ryan PJ, Harrison R, Blake GM, *et al.* Compliance with hormone replacement therapy (HT) after screening for postmenopausal osteoporosis. *Br J Obstet Gynaecol* 1992;99:325–8

8. Wallace WA, Price VH, Elliot CA, *et al.* Hormone replacement therapy acceptability to Nottingham postmenopausal women with a risk factor for osteoporosis. *J R Soc Med* 1990;83:699–701

9. Hartmann BW, Huber C. The mythology of hormone replacement therapy. *Br J Obstet Gynaecol* 1997;104:163–8

10. Albery N. The menopause in Japan – Konenki Jigoku. *Climacteric* 1999;2:160–1

11. Hughes CL, Cline JM, Williams JK, *et al.* Dietary soy phytoestrogens and the health of menopausal women; overview

and evidence of cardioprotection from studies in non-human primates. In Wren BG, ed. *Progress in the Management of the Menopause*. Carnforth, UK: Parthenon Publishing, 1996:12–17

12. Picherit C, Coxam V, Bennetau-Pelissero C, *et al*. Daidzein is more efficient than genistein in preventing ovariectomy induced bone loss in rats. *J Nutr* 2000;130:1675–81

13. Vincent A, Fitzpatrick LA. Soy isoflavones: are they useful in the menopause? *Mayo Clin Proc* 2000;75:1174–84

14. Simons LA, von Konigsmark M, Simons J, Celermajer DS. Phytoestrogens do not influence lipoprotein levels or endothelial function in healthy postmenopausal women. *Am J Cardiol* 2000;85:1297–301

15. Howes JB, Sullivan D, Lai N, *et al*. The effects of dietary supplementation with isoflavones from red clover on the lipoprotein profiles of postmenopausal women with mild to moderate hypercholesterolaemia. *Atherosclerosis* 2000;152:143–7

16. Dalais FS, Rice GE, Wahlqvist ML, *et al*. The effects of dietary phytoestrogens in postmenopausal women. *Climacteric* 1998;1:124–9

17. Scheiber MD, Rebar RW. Isoflavones and postmenopausal bone health; a viable alternative to estrogen therapy? *Menopause* 1999;6:233–41

18. Vincent A, Fitzpatrick LA. Soy isoflavones: are they useful in the menopause? *Mayo Clin Proc* 2000;75:1174–84

19. Albertazzi P, Pansini F, Bonaccorsi G, *et al*. The effect of dietary soy supplementation and phytoestrogen levels. *Obstet Gynecol* 1994;94:229–31

20. Quella SK, Loprinzi CL, Barton DL, et al. Evaluation of soy phytoestrogens for the treatment of hot flashes in breast cancer survivors: a North Central Cancer Treatment Group Trial. J Clin Oncol 2000;18:1068–74

21. Campbell S, Whitehead M. Estrogen therapy and the menopausal syndrome. Clin Obstet Gynaecol 1977;1:31–47

22. Davis SR. Phytoestrogen for menopausal symptoms? There's no good evidence that it's better than placebo. Br Med J 2001;323:354–5

23. Borelli F, Ernst E. Cimicifuga racemosa: a systemic review of its clinical effects. Eur J Clin Pharmacol 2002;58:235–41

24. Huntley A, Ernst E. A systematic review of the safety of black cohosh. Menopause 2003;10:58–64

25. Chenoy R, Hussain S, Tayob Y, et al. Effect of oral gamolenic acid from evening primrose oil on menopausal flushing. Br Med J 1994;19:501–3

26. Lee J. Osteoporosis reversal: the role of progesterone. Int Clin Nutr Rev 1990;10:384–9

27. Leonetti HB, Longo S, Anasti JN. Transdermal progesterone cream for vasomotor symptoms and postmenopausal bone loss. Obstet Gynecol 1999;94:225–8

28. Cooper A, Spencer C, Whitehead MI, et al. Systemic absorption of micronised progesterone from Progest cream in post menopausal women. Lancet 1998;351:1255–6

29. Wren BG, McFarland K, Edwards L, et al. Effect of sequential transdermal cream on endometrium, bleeding pattern, and

plasma progesterone levels in postmenopausal women. *Climacteric* 2000;3:155–60

30. Vickers M, Meade T, Darbyshire J. WISDOM: history and early demise – was it inevitable? *Climacteric* 2002;5:317–25

31. Shumaker SA, Legault C, Rapp SR, *et al.* Estrogen plus progestins and the incidence of dementia and mild cognitive impairment in postmenopausal women: the Women's Health Initiative Memory Study: a randomised controlled trial. *J Am Med Assoc* 2003;289:2651–62

Appendix

The following Tables list a selection of HT preparations available in the UK and USA.

Continuous combined HT preparations (CCEPT)

Trade names	Preparation	Active ingredient	Dose
Activella, Kliovance	tablet	estradiol 1 mg + norethisterone acetate 500 μg	1 tablet daily
Climesse	tablet	estradiol valerate 2 mg + norethisterone 700 μg	1 tablet daily
CombiPatch	patch	estradiol 50 μg/24 h + norethisterone acetate 0.14 mg/24 h	1 patch twice weekly
Elleste-Duet Conti, Kliofem, Nuvelle Continuous	tablet	estradiol 2 mg + norethisterone acetate 1 mg	1 tablet daily
Evorel Conti	patch	estradiol 50 μg/24 h + norethisterone acetate 170 μg/24 h	1 patch twice weekly
Femhrt	tablet	ethinylestradiol 5 μg + norethisterone acetate 1 mg	1 tablet daily
Femoston Conti	tablet	estradiol 1 mg + dydrogesterone 5 mg	1 tablet daily
FemSeven Conti	patch	ethinylestradiol 50 μg/24 h + levonorgestrel 25 μg/24 h	1 patch weekly
Indivina	tablet	estradiol valerate 1 mg + medroxyprogesterone acetate 2.5 mg (also 1 mg/5 mg and 2 mg/5 mg)	1 tablet daily
Livial	tablet	tibolone 2.5 mg	1 tablet daily
Premique, Prempro	tablet	conjugated equine estrogen 625 μg + medroxy-progesterone acetate 5 mg	1 tablet daily
Premfest	tablet	estradiol 1 mg + norgestimate 90 μg	1 tablet daily

Sequential HT preparations (CSEPT)

Trade names	Preparation	Active ingredient	Dose
Adgyn Combi	tablet	white tablet: estradiol 2 mg; pink tablet: estradiol 2 mg + norethisterone 1 mg	1 white tablet daily for 16 days, then 1 pink tablet for 12 days
Climagest	tablet	grey-blue tablet: estradiol valerate 1 mg (also 2 mg strength); white tablet: estradiol valerate 1 mg + norethisterone 1 mg	1 grey-blue tablet daily for 16 days, then 1 white tablet daily for 12 days
Cyclo-Progynova	tablet	beige tablet: estradiol valerate 1 mg; brown tablet: estradiol valerate 1 mg + levonorgestrel 250 μg (also 2 mg strength with estradiol valerate 2 mg + norgestrel 500 μg)	1 beige tablet daily for 11 days, then 1 brown tablet daily for 10 days, followed by a 7-day interval
Elleste-Duet	tablet	white tablet: estradiol 1 mg (also 2 mg strength); green tablet: estradiol 1 mg + norethisterone acetate 1 mg	1 white tablet daily for 16 days, then 1 green tablet daily for 12 days
Estracombi	patch	Estraderm TTS 50: estradiol 50 μg/24 h; Estragest TTS: estradiol 50 μg/24 h + norethisterone acetate 250 μg/24 h	1 Estraderm patch twice weekly for 2 weeks, then 1 Estragest patch twice weekly for 2 weeks
Estrapak 50	patch and tablet	patch: estradiol 50 μg/24 h; tablet: norethisterone acetate 1 mg	1 patch twice weekly and 1 tablet daily on days 15–26 of each 28-day cycle
Evorel Pak	patch and tablet	patch: estradiol 50 μg/24 h; tablet: norethisterone 1 mg	1 patch twice weekly and 1 tablet daily on days 15–26 of each 28-day cycle

continued

Sequential HT preparations (continued)

Trade names	Preparation	Active ingredient	Dose
Evorel Sequi	patch	Evorel 50: estradiol 50 μg/24 h; Evorel Conti: estradiol 50 μg/24 h + norethisterone 0.17 mg/24 h	1 Evoral 50 patch twice weekly for 2 weeks, then 1 Evorel Conti patch twice weekly for 2 weeks
Femapak	patch and tablet	patch: estradiol 40 μg/24 h (also 80 μg strength); tablet: dydrogesterone 10 mg	1 patch twice weekly and 1 tablet daily on days 15–28 of each 28-day cycle
Femoston	tablet	white tablet: estradiol 1 mg (also 2 mg strength); grey tablet: estradiol 1 mg + dydrogesterone 10 mg	1 white tablet daily for 14 days, then 1 grey tablet daily for 14 days
FemSeven Sequi	patch	phase I patch: estradiol 50 μg/24 h; phase II patch: estradiol 50 μg/24 h + levonorgestrel 25 μg/24 h	1 phase I patch weekly for 2 weeks, then 1 phase II patch weekly for 2 weeks
NovoFem	tablet	red tablet: estradiol 1 mg; white tablet: estradiol 1 mg + norethisterone acetate 1 mg	1 red tablet daily for 16 days, then 1 white tablet for 12 days
Nuvelle	tablet	white tablet: estradiol valerate 2 mg; pink tablet: estradiol valerate 2 mg + levonorgestrel 75 μg	1 white tablet daily for 16 days, then 1 pink tablet daily for 12 days
Nuvelle TS	patch	phase I patch: estradiol 80 μg/24 h; phase II patch: estradiol 50 μg/24 h + levonorgestrel 20 μg/24 h	1 phase I twice weekly for 2 weeks, then 1 phase II twice weekly for 2 weeks

continued

Sequential HT preparations (continued)

Trade names	Preparation	Active ingredient	Dose
Premique Cycle	tablet	white tablet: conjugated equine estrogen 625 μg; green tablet: conjugated equine estrogen 625 μg + medroxyprogesterone acetate 10 mg	1 white tablet daily for 14 days, then 1 green tablet daily for 14 days
Prempak-C	tablet	maroon tablet: conjugated equine estrogen 625 μg; brown tablet: norgestrel 150 μg (also 1.25 mg tablet)	1 maroon tablet daily and 1 brown tablet daily on days 17–28 of each 28-day cycle
Premphase	tablet	maroon tablet: conjugated equine estrogen 625 μg; blue tablet: conjugated equine estrogen 625 μg + medroxyprogesterone acetate 5 mg	1 maroon tablet daily for 14 days, then 1 blue tablet daily for 14 days
Tridestra	tablet	white tablet: estradiol valerate 2 mg; blue tablet: estradiol valerate 2 mg + medroxy-progesterone acetate 20 mg; yellow tablet: inactive	1 white tablet daily for 70 days, then 1 blue tablet daily for 14 days, then 1 yellow tablet daily for 7 days
Trisequens	tablet	blue tablet: estradiol 2 mg; white tablet: estradiol 2 mg + norethisterone acetate 1 mg; red tablet: estradiol 1 mg	1 blue tablet daily, then 1 tablet daily in sequence

Estrogen-only HT preparations

Trade names	Preparation	Active ingredient	Dose
Adgyn Estro	tablet	estradiol 2 mg	2 mg daily
Aerodiol	nasal spray	estradiol 150 μg/spray	I spray in each nostril daily at same time, either continuously or for 21–28 days followed by 2–7 days treatment-free. Number of sprays can be 1–4/day
Climara, Estraderm MX, Estraderm TTS, Evorel, Vivelle	patch	estradiol 25, 50, 75 or 100 μg/24 h	I patch twice weekly
Climaval, Progynova	tablet	estradiol valerate 1 or 2 mg	1–2 mg daily
Dermestril	patch	estradiol 25, 50 or 100 μg/24 h	I patch every 3–4 days
Dermestril-Septem	patch	estradiol 25, 50 or 75 μg/24 h	I patch once a week
Elleste-Solo	tablet	estradiol 1 or 2 mg	1–2 mg daily
Elleste-Solo MX, Fematrix	patch	estradiol 40 or 80 μg/24 h	I patch twice weekly
FemPatch, Progynova TS	patch	estradiol 50 or 100 μg/ 24 h	I patch once a week
FemSeven	patch	estradiol 50, 75 or 100 μg/24 h	I patch once a week
Harmogen	tablet	estropipate 1.5 mg	1.5–3 mg daily
Hormonin	tablet	estradiol 600 μg + estriol 270 μg + estrone 1.4 mg	1–2 tablets daily

continued

Estrogen-only HT preparations (continued)

Trade names	Preparation	Active ingredient	Dose
Menorest	patch	estradiol 37.5, 50 or 75 μg/24 h	1 patch twice weekly
Oestrogel	gel	estradiol 64-dose pump	2 measures (estradiol 1.5 mg) daily
Ovestin	tablet	estriol 1 mg	0.5–3 mg daily for up to 1 month, then 0.5–1 mg daily*
Premarin	tablet	conjugated equine estrogen 625 μg or 1.25 mg	0.625–1.25 mg daily
Sandrena	gel	estradiol 500 μg or 1 mg	0.5–1.5 mg daily
Zumenon	tablet	estradiol 1 mg or 2 mg	1–4 mg daily

*short-term treatment for genitourinary symptoms

Progestogen-only preparations suitable for HT

Trade names	Preparation	Active ingredient	Dose
Adgyn Medro	tablet	medroxyprogesterone acetate 5 mg	10 mg daily for days 15–28 of each 28-day estrogen HT cycle
Duphaston HT	tablet	dydrogesterone 10 mg	10 mg daily on days 15–28 of each 28-day estrogen HT cycle
Micronor HT	tablet	norethisterone 1 mg	1 mg daily on days 15–26 of each 28-day estrogen HT cycle
Mirena*	intrauterine device	levonorgestrel 20 μg	20 μg daily
Provera	tablet	medroxyprogesterone acetate 10 mg	10 mg daily for days 15–28 of each 28-day estrogen HT cycle

* Not yet licensed for HT in most countries

Chart for determining body mass index

Height (m)	Weight (kg) 45	50	55	60	65	70	75	80	85	90	95	100	105	110	115	120	125	130	135
1.4	23	26	28	31	33	36	38	41	43	46	48	51	54	56	59	61	64	66	69
1.425	22	25	27	30	32	34	37	39	42	44	47	49	52	54	57	59	62	64	66
1.45	21	24	26	29	31	33	36	38	40	43	45	48	50	52	55	57	59	62	64
1.475	21	23	25	28	30	32	34	37	39	41	44	46	48	51	53	55	57	60	62
1.5	20	22	24	27	29	31	33	36	38	40	42	44	47	49	51	53	56	58	60
1.525	19	21	24	26	28	30	32	34	37	39	41	43	45	47	49	52	54	56	58
1.55	19	21	23	25	27	29	31	33	35	37	40	42	44	46	48	50	52	54	56
1.575	18	20	22	24	26	28	30	32	34	36	38	40	42	44	46	48	50	52	54
1.6	18	20	21	23	25	27	29	31	33	35	37	39	41	43	45	47	49	51	53
1.625	17	19	21	23	25	27	28	30	32	34	36	38	40	42	44	45	47	49	51
1.65	17	18	20	22	24	26	28	29	31	33	35	37	39	40	42	44	46	48	50
1.675	16	18	20	21	23	25	27	29	30	32	34	36	37	39	41	43	45	46	48
1.7	16	17	19	21	22	24	26	28	29	31	33	35	36	38	40	42	43	45	47
1.725	15	17	18	20	22	24	25	27	29	30	32	34	35	37	39	40	42	44	45
1.75	15	16	18	20	21	23	24	26	28	29	31	33	34	36	38	39	41	42	44
1.775	14	16	17	19	21	22	24	25	27	29	30	32	33	35	37	38	40	41	43
1.8	14	15	17	19	20	22	23	25	26	28	29	31	32	34	35	37	39	40	42
1.825	14	15	17	18	20	21	23	24	26	27	29	30	32	33	35	36	38	39	41
1.85	13	15	16	18	19	20	22	23	25	26	28	29	31	32	34	35	37	38	39
1.875	13	14	16	17	18	20	21	23	24	26	27	28	30	31	33	34	36	37	38
1.9	12	14	15	17	18	19	21	22	24	25	26	28	29	30	32	33	35	36	37
1.925	12	13	15	16	18	19	20	22	23	24	26	27	28	30	31	32	34	35	36
1.95	12	13	14	16	17	18	20	21	22	24	25	26	28	29	30	32	33	34	36
1.975	12	13	14	15	17	18	19	21	22	23	24	26	27	28	29	31	32	33	35
2.0	11	13	14	15	16	18	19	20	21	23	24	25	26	28	29	30	31	33	34

Body mass index expressed as kg /m². Light grey shading, obese; dark grey, over-weight; white, normal

Index